A PATHWAY TO RECOVER Y~~

Regenesis

Diabetes
Arthritis
Obesity
Fatigue
Fibromyalgia
Inflammation
Digestive Issues
Heartburn
General Poor Health

DR. GARRY COLLINS

The opinions expressed in this manuscript are solely the opinions of the author and do not represent the opinions or thoughts of the publisher. The author has represented and warranted full ownership and/or legal right to publish all the materials in this book.

Regenesis
All Rights Reserved.
Copyright © 2015 Dr. Garry Collins
v5.0

Cover Photo © 2015 thinkstockphotos.com. All rights reserved - used with permission.
Butterflies by Dr. Jackie Alvarez Maxwell

This book may not be reproduced, transmitted, or stored in whole or in part by any means, including graphic, electronic, or mechanical without the express written consent of the publisher except in the case of brief quotations embodied in critical articles and reviews.

Outskirts Press, Inc.
http://www.outskirtspress.com

ISBN: 978-1-4787-4578-5

Outskirts Press and the "OP" logo are trademarks belonging to Outskirts Press, Inc.

PRINTED IN THE UNITED STATES OF AMERICA

DISCLAIMER

The ideas opinions and concepts in this book are intended to be used for educational purposes only. This book and the REGENESIS program and its recommendations have not been evaluated by the FDA or any other governmental agency. It is not meant to diagnose or treat any disease, condition or illness. Reading a book is not a substitute for quality healthcare issued by a competent physician. I have done my best to ensure the information is accurate. At the writing of this book, I did not hold any degree in clinical nutrition or nutritional counseling. The author and the publisher of this book cannot assume responsibility for any loss or risk, personal or otherwise, that is incurred as a direct or indirect consequence of the use or the application of any of the information in this book. Discontinuing medications is a serious thing and should be monitored by your doctor. If you have a disease or condition, you should have full medical clearance from a qualified health care professional before exercising or making significant dietary changes. Dietary changes can cause significant changes in blood sugar and insulin needs for diabetics. Monitoring blood sugar levels and blood pressure are wise things to do particularly if you are a diabetic or have other health challenges and make significant changes to your diet. Some vitamins and nutritional supplements can interfere with medicines. Addition of supplements to a daily health regimen should be done with the assistance of your health care provider. If you have a medical problem you should seek the advice of a competent medical provider.

Mentioning organizations, companies, or products does not imply endorsement by the author or the publisher. As of the writing of this book, there are no current endorsements of this work for the author or the publisher.

All websites given in this book were accurate at the time of printing.

Special Thanks

THERE ARE SO many people to thank for their various talents and knowledge in helping me to accomplish one of my goals in life. First and foremost, my long time mate of thirty years, Donna. She keeps me grounded and gives me a viewpoint that I don't always see. Her love, companionship, and honesty is priceless and I am so blessed to have found her. To my parents, Paul and Geneva Collins who "raised me right" and taught me the importance of self-reliance and honesty. To my brothers and sisters Barry, Cathy, Danny and Brenda; that never let me forget where I came from. To all of my mentors especially Dr. Joel Wallach, Dr. John Brimhall and Dr. Paul Goldberg. My doctor friends from school: Dr. Gary Barker, Dr. Jackie Alvarez Maxwell, Dr. Wendy Rod, Dr. Chris Horner, Dr. Jerry Baker, and Dr. Bruce Deutsch. I can call any of them anytime for any reason; that is a priceless resource. A special thanks to my patients that have allowed me to be a part of their lives and to grow and learn from their experiences. To my staff Lorrie Harrison, Joy France, who keep me from the minutia and the mountain of paper that I so dislike in business. They constantly support me in my many endeavors, I could not practice without them. To Dr. Linda Petrie, Bob and Debra Ashcraft, for their input. A big thanks to Inge Terrill for her skills, knowledge and all of the long hours spent helping me with the final edit. Much gratitude to my geek friend Amy Adams. To my Attorney and long-time friend Kendall Clay, his work allowed me to pursue my goal of becoming a Dr. of Chiropractic, it's a long story. I have three special friends I have known since high school; they had a profound influence on the early trajectory of my life. I love them like brothers, Kim Love, Paul Weeks, and John O'Conner. I have been blessed over the years to have made many friends. There is no way I could mention them all.

BUTTERFLIES

To me the metamorphosis of the butterfly is symbolic of the long journey to recover one's health. I love to photograph them. I have chosen the butterfly as the symbol of the REGENESIS program. There is an incredible butterfly in all of us waiting for its wings.

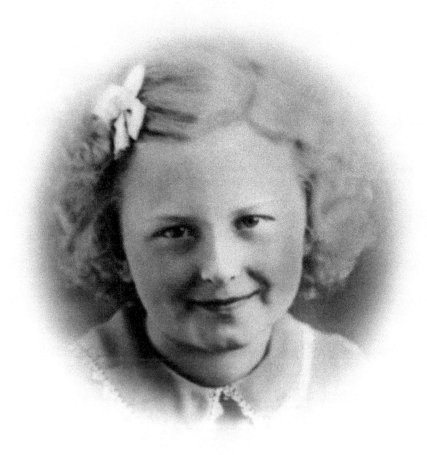

This beautiful young girl was born Sept. 4th, 1930. She did not know at the time of this photograph that she would live the last fifty years of her life with sugar diabetes. Sadly, during the writing of this book, she passed away (Dec. 23, 2012). Although she never knew it, this book was inspired by her and the struggles she endured at the end of her life. This is a picture of my mother. She died at home from the complications of diabetes in the loving arms of her family. This little girl became the most wonderful mother to her 5 children and a devoted wife of 64 years to our father. She was honest, kind, loving and fearless when she needed to be.

We miss her so much.
Geneva Aldeen Collins
This book is dedicated to her memory.
May she rest in eternal peace.

A Word About Diets

I WANT TO be perfectly frank about something right from the start. THERE IS NO DIET THAT WILL WORK FOR EVERYONE!! There are so many factors that can affect the results that people get. There must be a thousand different diet books in the book stores now. What makes the dietary component of this program any different? The REGENESIS program is not just a diet, it is a health program. This program is a starting point. It is meant to make you aware of the fact that it takes more than just a diet to get healthy. It requires awareness, a constant quest for knowledge, and a willingness to work on that new knowledge. Health is a lifetime process.

We live in a toxic environment! There are chemicals all around us, in our water, air, homes, clothing, beauty products, air fresheners, and in our cars. Our processed convenient food supply is laced with chemicals. We are surrounded by emotionally toxic and negative people. I think you know what I mean here.

Have you ever known a couple that tried the Atkins Diet and got vastly different results? I had an overweight couple that did this, he lost 90 lbs., she lost 10 lbs. They were eating virtually the same thing so how could the outcome be so different? This is an example of what I am talking about. It could be genetics, food allergies, malabsorption issues, different mental attitudes, lack of commitment on someone's part, or varying degrees of physical activities. I can go on and on.

Some people don't like vegetables, some people don't like meats, or they are opposed to eating animals for philosophical or religious reasons. Some people don't have the resolve or the peer support they need to be successful. So will the REGENESIS program "work" for everyone? NO. But it will work for a lot of people, especially for people who are truly looking for a different approach, an opposing view from the ever changing current but questionable health and dietary dogma.

If you are the type of person that needs a guideline to help you stay on target, I would highly recommend the REGENESIS work book, sold separately.

If the REGENESIS program doesn't work for you, keep trying until you find one that does. Your health is worth it!

Contents

*	Introduction	1
1.	How Did We Get So Sick?	7
2.	Water	29
3.	Wheat	43
4.	Sugars	61
5.	Oils, Fats, and Cholesterol	82
6.	Food Additives	108
7.	Chemical Madness	125
8.	Warning Lights	137
9.	Supplementation	151
10.	Movement	165
11.	Leftovers	176
12.	Eating Guidelines	199
13.	In Conclusion	213
*	REGENESIS Food List	217
*	REGENESIS Program Plan Summary	219
*	Recipes	221
*	Appendix	232
*	Works Cited	235
*	Index	257

Introduction

I WAS EIGHT years old when my mother told me she had sugar diabetes. I did not fully understand what that meant. I found myself crying on the back steps because I was afraid that my mother was going to die. Like any good mother, she came to my side hugged me and assured me that she was going to be okay and that all she had to do was watch what she ate. Fifty years later my fear was validated.

In December of 2012, my family and I were going through all of our family picture albums as we needed to find pictures of my mother. She died two days before Christmas from the complications of fifty years of living with type 2 diabetes. It was a somber time but provided us time together as a family and we found some levity in the pictures our family had collected for over 65 years. We all commented on how much healthier we all were when we were kids and how skinny everyone was.

As youngsters we played in the creeks, we drank raw milk every day, and played outside until dark even in the winter time. We worked in the hayfields and tobacco fields even as pre-teenagers. We rarely had to go to the doctor and if we did it was usually because we had a broken bone or needed stitches. None of the neighborhood kids were overweight. Stark contrast to what I see in young folks today.

While looking through all of those pictures, I found a couple of my high school annuals. We only had one or two class mates that were overweight. In the mornings before I go to work, I stop at a local convenience store to get a small cup of coffee and what I witness there is sobering. I watch our high school kids mixed in with people going to work purchasing the brightly packaged poison that is slowly killing them. The kids all seem to have acne and or they are overweight and in some cases both. The adults going to work look as if they can barely open their eyes, they all look so tired and worn down.

The evidence is mounting and more and more voices are sounding alarms about the health of our nation. We are more and more unhealthy, obese, and infirmed than at any other time in our history. Just a few years ago diabetes was a disease of aging it was called adult onset diabetes, that term is no longer valid. We are seeing type 2 diabetes in our teenagers; now more than 168,000 people under the age of twenty have the disease [1] Our current health care model, our governmental agencies, and our food manufacturing institutions are failing us miserably. What is it going to take to wake us up? There is so much confusion, mis-information and fraud taking place in our food and drug industry. More drugs for more diseases, new drugs for emerging diseases like Alzheimer's disease.

Fifty years ago, Alzheimer's was not in the lexicon of mainstream America, obesity and diabetes were not rampant like today.[2] Incidences of cancer seem to be exploding in spite of the billions of dollars being poured into finding the cure.[3] Heart disease and cardiovascular disease is not in check even though billions of dollars are being spent on statin drugs, dietary interventions, and invasive heart procedures. [4]

Where is all of this disease and infirmity coming from? It only makes sense to me to look at things we all share in common. We all have to eat, drink, and breathe. Let's start there.

Our national food supply is so modified and adulterated by genetic engineering, hybridization, preservatives, artificial sweeteners, packaging, and refinement. Our obsession with sugary laden soft drinks, so called power drinks, candy, packaged cakes, donuts, boxed cereals, and other junk foods is well documented in the bottom lines of the manufacturer's ledgers. The average American consumes over 150 lbs. of sugar a year. (5) There are over 320,000 processed foods in America and over a quarter-million fast food restaurants competing for your business. (6)

We drink water from chemically produced plastic bottles, our wells and springs are polluted from over one hundred years of chemical production and pollution. Our air is polluted both inside and outside of our homes.

I have been on this band wagon for over ten years, many others on the wagon long before me. Now we are hearing and seeing a trickle of the evidence showing up on the mainstream media outlets. Many brave doctors are stepping out of the box and writing books. Research has been done that refutes much of the standard treatments that are being given in doctor's offices all around the country.

To me the biggest fraud is the cholesterol lie. I'm not saying that cholesterol is something that should be ignored I'm saying that its role as a health marker is being mis-represented to the public.(7) Blaming cholesterol for disease is like blaming firemen for fires, or rats for landfills.

Observing all of this insanity from my small office in rural Virginia, has made me a cynical contrarian as the words in this book will clearly demonstrate. I don't know how everyone can't see past the smoke that is being blown at us about how great American health care is. According to recent CIA documentation for the year 2013, we are 51st in longevity of industrialized nations.(8) Our infant mortality is among the worst of the industrialized nations.(9) We have the most expensive health care in the world, that much is true. In defense of our health care institutions, we do have excellent trauma care in America. Now even if you do not believe in our health care delivery methods, you are going to be forced to pay for it, and fined by the IRS (the largest collection agency in the world) if you fail to do your part. So much for freedom in health care, I can only imagine what is next. The camel has his nose under the tent.

After careful consideration, it seems to me that the best health insurance is a pro-active approach from an individual perspective; simply put, take care of yourself. Use healthcare providers for information but make positive changes so as not to create dependency on chemical medications for the answers. This is difficult to do considering the massive amount of conflicting information that is available. How can we sort through what is truth and what is fiction? What works for one person may not work for another. This is due in large part to what I call "biochemical individuality". If you are truly observant, and are willing to make adjustments to your diet and lifestyle, true health can be accomplished.

There are some basic truths that apply to everyone, and it is the goal of this book to point out some of those truths just to get you started in the right direction. Many of these truths will go against what you have been taught by watching your TV's, or what you have read in so called "health" magazines, or ridiculous ten second sound bites you've heard on the radio.

The REGENESIS program is something that happened by default. The more ill health I witnessed in my patients, the more I read about the true causes of diseases, the more I began to speak out to my patients about their lifestyle choices. Some things were becoming very evident to me; I couldn't understand why everyone else couldn't see the obvious reasons for their health problems. I began writing one page "reports" to hand to my patients on particular issues. I accumulated several different ones and eventually stapled them together. They varied from some reasonable dietary changes to fibromyalgia, from some facts on the dangers and the adverse effects of Aspartame, to the truth about cholesterol. I eventually developed a "packet" of information. One day I got the bright idea that instead of trying to talk to my patients during my busy work schedule, I would teach a "class" on the things I wanted to talk to them about.

Little did I know of the dramatic effect this "class" was going to have on some of my patients. From this humble start the REGENESIS program has evolved. This book is yet another step in the evolution of this program. While this book contains information from books various websites and scientific studies, it also contains a lot of my personal opinions based on my experiences as a health care provider.

I know by experience that there are a lot of people that would make the right choices if they were given some simple truths to start with and to build on. I know my mother would have been one of them. Fifty years ago if she had known what I know now and what was going to happen to her and her family in the last 12 years of her life, she would have absolutely made the proper choices. She loved us all very much and it was humbling for her and for us to provide the level of care she needed especially in the last three years of her life. She was blessed to have a husband and children that had the ability to care for her needs. I am so proud to be a part of a family that is responsible, caring, and hard working. None of us could have done this alone. Not all families are this fortunate, but unfortunately, our story is not unique. After observing my mother's hardships I particularly hate what has happened in regards to diabetes and the treatment recommendations to the millions of diabetics in America.

There are a host of diseases and conditions spawned by a diabetic lifestyle: hypertension, kidney problems, heart disease, poor circulation, depression, Alzheimer's disease, peripheral neuropathy, and others. Amazingly, there are some basic nutritional truths that most of the diabetics I know have never heard. I have tried my best to boil these truths down into some very basic concepts that are steeped in common sense.

I realize that there is no one answer for every person or condition, I am just attempting to open our collective eyes to these basic truths about health. Agree or disagree, the fact is that America is sick and getting worse by most objective measurements. I would encourage everyone to take control of their own health, and reduce the dependency on the over-priced, over utilized sub-standard "health" care system we have. By all means, use the trauma and emergency care when it is necessary. However, when it comes to health, you are on your own. Doctors, hospitals, and our current health care system are centered around screenings for diseases, disease management, and expensive interventions, not "health" care.

I have boxed out some paragraphs of my actual clinical experiences in the book that help to make what I am telling you more real. I have also included some of the books that have led me to where I am today so that you may see what I see.

It is my hope that Americans will start participating and creating their own good health by reading and listening to some of these modern day health prophets.

I wish you well on your journey,
I wish you a new beginning.
I wish you a
"REGENESIS"

1

How Did We Get So Sick?

"If you don't know where you are going, any road will get you there."
Lewis Carroll (Alice In Wonderland)

GENETICISTS AGREE THAT humans have the genetic potential to live 120 years or more. In Genesis 6:3 it says: "Man is of the flesh and he shall live 120 years." Why are we as Americans not meeting our genetic potential for longevity and health? There are many reasons that people are not living quality healthful lives today. Granted we are living much longer than we did in 1900, mainly because of improvements in water quality, sterilization procedures, and managing bacterial infections that once killed millions of people. Now many of us are suffering and then dying prematurely due to diseases caused by our modern conveniences and the gradual but profound shift in lifestyle they have created.

Most likely you are reading my book now because of the "status quo" in America. It is likely that you have been eating the Standard American Diet (SAD) based on the food pyramid. You are also probably living a highly stressed life, not resting or exercising enough, watching too much television, and not engaging in your own well-being. You have a family doctor, or in some cases, several doctors, whose advice you have been following for years. If you are the typical American over forty years of age, you are probably taking multiple over the counter and or prescription medications.

It seems the more conveniences that we enjoy and the more "civilized" we become, the sicker we become. We have moved away from preparing healthy foods and drinking healthy water. We are not enjoying family and leisure time. There has been a gradual movement away from our spiritual and religious institutions. We have moved toward adulterated packaged foods and we eat too much fast food. We trust chemically treated tap water or water in plastic bottles. We think that medical technologies and medicines made from chemicals give us health.

In most families, both parents are working (if both parents are present), and often at very stressful jobs. A lot of people seemingly worship their computers and personal communication devices. There are cell towers and Wi-Fi networks everywhere, microwave ovens in our kitchens, and televisions in every room of our house and in our cars. Our bodies are bombarded by electro-magnetic forces (EMF) daily, a problem that very few people know about. Industry in America and other countries introduce hundreds, if not thousands, of new chemical compounds to our water, air, and food every year. We are drowning in "civilization" and the "technology" that has created all of our modern conveniences. As the pace of our lives speed up, there seems to be less time to engage in the personal responsibility for our health, in spite of the time created by the so-called conveniences we enjoy.

Is it just me, or does there seem to be a pill for everything these days? Americans take most of the world's drugs.[1] If drugs made you healthy, the people taking the most drugs would be the healthiest, we know that simply is not the case. There is plenty of blame to go around for our poor health as a nation, such as our health institutions, our doctors, the media, our food industry, the government, and others. Ultimately, we as individuals must assume the bulk of the responsibility. It is not up to large corporations, your doctor, or your government to take care of your health. It's up to you! This will be a recurrent theme in the following pages.

See if you can relate to the following example: It's up in the morning after sleeping with the aid of a sleeping pill. Then a bath or shower with chlorinated and fluoridated water using soaps, shampoos and body washes that are laden with toxic chemicals. From there it's to the kitchen where the prescription medications are kept in a pill organizer for convenience. We pour ourselves some highly processed boxed cereal laced with chemicals and sugars into a bowl and drown it with some highly processed milk, along with more sugar. Then it's chased down the gullet with some coffee, soda, chocolate milk, or sweet juice.

Off to our jobs that most of us do not enjoy, working for people that we do not like, and dealing with the public that is more and more demanding all the time. Anger, frustration, and stress escalates through the day until we are finally off work and headed home. Too tired to cook, it is much easier to stop by the pizza place and pick up a couple of pizzas along with a bottle or two of soda, one regular, one diet. We head for home behind some slow poke driving 35 mph and hitting every stop light. After the stress from our work day and road rage, we gulp down supper. At night, we sit in front of the television, snacking on popcorn or some other unhealthy food until bedtime. Just before turning in, we take our Ambien or Lunesta to help us sleep and the cycle starts all over again.

Does this or part of this sound familiar to you? Do you know someone like this? Are you like this? Does this sound like quality living?

Notice in this scenario, there is no mention of drinking pure water, or cooking a quality meal from scratch with organic foods. No mention is made of working at a job or trade that one really enjoys alongside people that are of like mind, even if the pay was a little less. No quality vitamin regimen is being followed. No thought is given to taking just ten minutes to reflect on how good your life is, through either prayer or meditation. Also absent in our little story is the time for a brisk walk in the fresh air and sunshine. Time around the kitchen table as a family is either limited or non-existent, because one of the children and the soccer mom are away to yet another sporting event. It's no wonder we only live a little more than 70 years in this country.

In the early 1900's, America was evolving from the horse and buggy to the automobile. There were wooden sidewalks, Sears and Roebuck catalogues, and modern appliances being developed. An industrial boom was in full swing. Oil and petroleum was becoming big business because of the changing infrastructure caused by the switch from horse and buggies to automobiles. At the forefront of that movement in America was the Rockefellers (Standard Oil). It was during this time that several health care ideologies were evolving including naturopathy, osteopathy, allopathy (medical doctors), chiropractic, homeopathy, and eclectic medicine.

In the early 1900's, the allopathic (MD) colleges and universities, created a powerful alliance with the petroleum and chemical (drug) industry, with financial incentives from the very wealthy Rockefellers and Carnegies.[2] A major power shift occurred in the politics of health care. As a result, wonderful healing arts like naturopathy, homeopathy, eclectic medicine and chiropractic, were crowded out of mainstream health. Any healers other than the allopathic doctors (MD's and osteopaths) were deemed charlatans and quacks. It is during this time that the "modern era" of health care began. Drugs began flowing like water and the flood continues today. Americans are drowning in prescription drugs.

Americans are drowning in prescription drugs.

Modern medicine really made its ascent past the other evolving health care models with help from the American Medical Association, the Rockefellers and Carnegies after the Flexner Report of 1910, also called the "Carnegie Foundation Bulletin Number Four". This report supported by big money from The Rockefeller Foundation, was designed to "weed out" substandard medical schools. While no doubt, there needed to be some standards set at that time for medical institutions, the effects on other healthcare disciplines (from that time forward labeled alternative) were devastating. Abraham Flexner was not a medical educator, or a physician, he believed only in the science of the day and anything not based in that science was invalid to him.

Just a reminder here about the science of the day; on Dec. 14th, 1799, the current "science" of blood-letting contributed to the death of our first president George Washington. The doctors took several pints of blood from him thinking it would heal him; it killed him at age 67. Current science is _always_ changing and subject to skepticism as well as humility.

Any schools that offered training in courses without the backing of scientific research like phototherapy, eclectic medicine (the use of medicinal herbs especially influenced by American Indian traditions), homeopathy, naturopathy or electromagnetic field therapy, were instructed to discontinue these classes. Schools that did not comply were told they would lose their accreditation and underwriting support. These schools either complied or shut down. (3)

The Flexner report along with the strong influence of the Rockefeller Foundation began to gradually eliminate all other schools of the healing arts. It also resulted in closing of schools that taught herbal medicine or manipulative therapies. This gave a strong advantage in the markets of the day to the allopathic schools (MD's). Medical schools affiliated with universities based in the scientific models of the day survived the "Sword of Damocles" that was created by the Flexner report.(4) Big money influence and politics wins again. Does this sound familiar?

In the time between 1848 and the mid 1920's, through various legislative medical practice acts, the allopathic medical profession (MD's) eventually became the overseers of our nation's health institutions and hospitals. This power grab, combined with the money and influence of the Rockefellers and Carnegies, and an emerging pharmaceutical industry, pushed other health disciplines out of the mainstream. As a result, the modern, drug based, reductionist (all problems can be solved by reducing things to their smallest parts) healthcare system that we have today was born. There are almost one million medical doctors in America today. This is due in large part to Abraham Flexner's work that was supported by two very wealthy and influential foundations so long ago.

The following lines are from an article about the Flexner Report written by Thomas P. Duffy in the *Yale Journal of Biology and Medicine, Sept. 2011; 84 (3):269-276* :

"…The discontent with doctor's errors, doctor's silence, doctor's experimentation, and the crass monetary orientation of the profession is legion. The profession appears to be losing its soul at the same time its body is clothed in a luminous garment of scientific knowledge.

This is especially ironic because the Teutonic heritage that provided the template for Flexner's plan also contains a cautionary message for him, for his circle and for all of us (MD's). It is the tale of Faust and the irresistible allure of knowledge in exchange for one's soul." [5]

Had Flexner's work, funded by the Rockefellers and the Carnegies, not occurred, the allopathic model, along with homeopathy, chiropractic, eclectic medicine, naturopathy, and osteopathy could have potentially evolved and integrated into a very diverse national health care system. This system could have been the envy of the world. Americans would have had all of these systems co-existing for the benefit of patients. Patients could pick and choose what works and does not work. This would have created innovation and competition and kept the costs of being healthy low; this is a free market approach. Now patients need to have permission from the gate keepers (their MD) if they want to see a chiropractor and have it paid for by their insurance. Naturopathy and homeopathy have been reduced to alternatives that are hard to find and are usually not covered by any types of health insurance.

Between 1950 and 1960, for insurance reimbursement reasons, the Osteopathic profession gave in to financial pressures and abandoned the "rule of the artery" upon which their original philosophy was founded [6]. Now for the most part, osteopaths are just medical doctors with a different suffix to their professional names (DO). The great old line "OMT" (Osteopathic Manipulative Therapy) osteopaths are all gone; a real tragedy. I feel certain that Dr. Andrew Still, the founder of osteopathy, has rolled over in his grave.

Two hundred and twenty five thousand Americans die every year of negligence at the hand of our modern health care system, making it the number three leading cause of death in America, some estimates are even higher![7] Three thousand Americans died on 9-11 and as a result, America went to war. Over a ten year period, 1.06 million people died in America from adverse drug reactions.[8] During the ten years of the Viet-Nam war, at least 56,000 Americans lost their lives in the jungles of southeast Asia. Our country was in turmoil, there were riots everywhere, including the Kent State massacre. Almost a quarter of a million Americans are killed by our health care system EVERY YEAR and no one goes to jail.[9] Have you seen all the drug commercials and the corresponding legal suits for some of those drugs on mainstream media? Where is the public outcry? Where is the media?

Americans spend more on healthcare and drugs than all other nations combined. Yet a recent study reveals that America is 51st out of 222 countries in longevity, close to the very bottom of industrialized nations [10]. People living in Greece, Jordan, and Bosnia outlive us. Out of the 222 countries in the study, most of them are third world countries. We are among the worst when it comes to infant mortality among industrialized nations.[11] We are more obese and sicker as a nation now than at any time in our modern history. Is this what we get for all the money we pay for health care? We would not accept these poor results at these high costs in any other profession. You would not pay the highest price for a roofer, auto mechanic, or a builder with results like this. Now, through *The Affordable Health Care Act,* we are all going to be forced, by legislation, to pay for it, and fined if we do not comply!

This major shift in our lifestyles began during the industrial revolution. The pace of our lives started to speed up and the effects on our personal health, as well as our national health, has been insidious and costly. Take a good look at our diseases. I can't name one of our top diseases in this country that is really on the decline.

Billions of dollars have been thrown at finding cures for diseases by organizations like the American Cancer Society, Relay for Life, Muscular Dystrophy Association, March of Dimes, The United Way, and seemingly hundreds of others just like them. Some charities have excessive and questionable administrative fees. A recent article on the pink breast cancer awareness attire worn by NFL players reports that only 8% of the money from that campaign actually goes to cancer research.[12] Huge amounts of government funded (taxpayer) dollars are also being spent on research. Almost all of the research is looking for that magic chemical bullet (patentable of course). So much money is being spent trying to win the "wars" against our diseases, but it's not working. We are not winning the "wars" against any major disease that I can see, especially diabetes and Alzheimer's disease.

We are not winning the "wars" against any major disease that I can see, especially diabetes and Alzheimer's disease.

Should we continue on this futile path or should we change course? Chemistry and the chemicals of civilization have contributed to our diseases like cancer, Parkinson's disease, multiple sclerosis (MS), cardiovascular disease, diabetes, arthritis, lupus, fibromyalgia, and many others. We use chemicals on our foods, our seeds, cosmetics, and fabrics. Tons of chemicals are in our air and water. These chemicals contribute to our diseases, then we try to solve our health problems with more chemicals. Albert Einstein said: *"We can't solve problems by using the same kind of thinking we used when we created them"*.

Dr. Joel Wallach always points out that Albert Einstein died of a ruptured aortic aneurysm, which is caused by a simple copper deficiency. Veterinarians fixed this problem in turkeys decades ago simply by adding copper into their feeds. (13) One of the smartest men of all time died of a simple mineral deficiency. We don't let turkeys die of copper deficiencies, but aneurysms continue to kill humans every day. Icons like John Ritter and Conway Twitty also died from ruptured aneurysms.

The early signs of copper deficiencies are: premature gray hair, spider and/or varicose veins, hemorrhoids, and wrinkles.(14) Look at one of the pictures of Albert Einstein. In hindsight, who couldn't have seen that one coming?

I talk to patients about prevention and common sense things routinely in my office. We discuss removing many of the man-made chemicals from their homes. This includes chemicals and preservatives found in cleaning supplies, foods, cosmetics and body care products. We talk about eliminating processed, chemical laden foods and replacing them with high density, quality foods. We discuss hydration and bowel habits. Bowel function is an important indicator of general health. All parents know that 20 or 30 minutes after feeding a baby, they dirty up a diaper. That gastro-intestinal rhythm should remain for the rest of your life. Twenty to thirty minutes after eating, you should have a bowel movement! This is rare in America today as our food supply and our diets are so poor. Many of my patients have very poor bowel function. One of my favorite quotes is from Mischio Kushi (of macrobiotic fame) who died well before he turned 100 years old, he said, *"Americans have small stools and big hospitals."* (15)

Unfortunately, it has been my experience that it is easier to talk to most of these same patients about diet and lifestyle after they have had a serious health event. It goes back to that old saying, "When the student is ready, the teacher will appear". Another old saying is "You can lead a horse to water, but you can't make him drink". I have revised the last saying to "You can lead a horse to water, but you can't hold his head under but so long". I preach health to some patients until I am blue in the face. They are "drowning" in health problems. Some of them just don't get it, or they are unwilling to change regardless of the potential consequences of their diets and lifestyles.

I vividly remember a patient that at one time weighed 370 pounds. I predicted to him that if he did not change his ways dramatically, he would soon become a diabetic and that he was at risk of a heart attack. I warned him that his knees and back would not be able to carry his weight much longer. After ten years, he is now a diabetic, he has had a heart attack, two back surgeries and his knees hurt him all of the time. His MD has prescribed him a handful of drugs that he believes he has to take just to remain alive. Now he wants to talk about his health. It is so much harder and more expensive to help him now. Why can't we see the future consequences of our current actions? Tomorrow's health is determined by today's choices.

Tomorrow's health is determined by today's choices.

Just as I don't always know what motivates people to move in unhealthy directions, I can't know what motivates people to make a decision to recapture their health. Motivation is deeply personal and is never the same for everyone. Planting a seed of thought or hope is the only thing that I can do. The final decision to do something about one's health is up to the individual.

Some people are motivated by the loss of function and inability to do certain things they once enjoyed like golfing or biking. Maybe it is not being able to spend quality time with their children or grandchildren. Many patients just feel bad all the time. In many cases this is from their health problems and the medications they have been given by their doctors to manage their diseases and symptoms. Most folks are not even aware that they can change their health and will never make the effort. To me this is the greatest tragedy.

I named this chapter "How Did We Get So Sick?" for two reasons. Number one: How did we get so unhealthy as a nation? Number two: How did we get so sick and unhealthy as individuals? These two questions are different, but intimately connected. As a nation, we are influenced by the surrounding social norms, traditions, commercial advertising, fast-paced lifestyles, and so called progress. As individuals, we make decisions on lifestyle based on our personal beliefs and the influences of our families, peers, our choice of media, and the culture in which we live. This ultimately creates the health situations that we live with, good or bad.

I really believe that it takes understanding and commitment to make the necessary changes to be healthy. I have created an equation for success when it comes to recapturing health. Understanding + ongoing commitment = success (health), in short u+(oc) = s. There is an equation for you Einstein, well I digress.

uderstanding + ongoing commitment = success (health)
u+(oc) = s

If you stop and think about it, it requires effort to obtain food and drink whether it is good or bad. If people fully understood their choices and were motivated to change, it is not any more difficult to obtain these healthier options than it is to obtain the unhealthy ones. The effort is basically the same.

I hear this comment all the time, "It's so hard to buy good food." Really? It is not hard to find good food. It requires understanding where to buy good food and making a conscious effort to shop there, the physical task is the same. To me it's more unwillingness to change and make a lifetime commitment to that change, not because it's hard to buy or find good food. Our shopping and eating habits are well established and sometimes not easily changed because they have become comfortable. People need to get out of their comfort zone if they are ever going to change their health.

It is not hard to find good food.

Recently, while shopping at a local big box pet store, I couldn't help but notice that, like everywhere else, most of the people in there were overweight. We were standing next to a very nice couple both of them were considerably overweight (easily 600 lbs combined). They were reading labels and laboring over the correct dog food to purchase. I also noticed that their pet looked particularly slim, alert and healthy. It was very obvious to me that they did not spend nearly as much time laboring over food labels, or choice of food for themselves.

Since most us do not insure our pets, the veterinarians and pet food scientists have created perfect foods for our animals. We have almost doubled the life span of our pet dogs. Why is it that we don't seem to have a clue when it comes to human nutrition? We have been doing this reduced fat, grain based, low cholesterol food pyramid project for decades now. The food pyramid (the prudent diet), that has contributed so much to our poor health, took decades of lies and deception to create. A great book that goes into a lot of detail about this is- *Death by Food Pyramid,* by Dense Minger.[16] It is on my recommended reading list. In 1985, the National Heart, Lung and Blood Institute recommended cutting saturated fats and cholesterol from our diets and replacing them with multiple servings of grain based carbohydrates. (17) Since we started following the advice of all of these expert agencies, we are more obese, have more heart disease, diabetes, cancer, and are more unhealthy now than ever before in our history.

> "The USDA's seven-food group pyramid has been a failure right out of the chute! The same people who express dismay at the fattening of American children put six to eleven servings of carbohydrates at the base and flagship feature of the seven food pyramid! The seven-food group pyramid was designed for high-energy output athletes who can burn 5,000 calories per day, not for the average grade school student and the data entry guy.
> If you want to make pigs fat give them carbohydrate! If you want to make cattle fat give them carbohydrate! If you want to make Americans fat give them the seven-food group pyramid!" (18)
>
> Dr. Joel Wallach, and Ma Lan MD.

With quality animal foods, our dogs and cats get perfect food with every bite. Humans eat highly processed non-nutritious, microwaveable, chemical laden, dead but fast foods. Maybe we should adopt the system used by the pet animal industry and use common sense nutrition first, instead of medicines.

Maybe we should adopt example given to us by the pet animal industry and use common sense nutrition first, instead of medicines.

There are so many topics to discuss, so much argument over who or what is right, so much mis-information out there, that it is seemingly impossible to know what to do or who to believe. With the REGENESIS program, there are basic foundational principles that apply to everyone: elimination of wheat and wheat products, avoiding soft drinks of all kinds, drinking pure water, eliminating refined sugar and excessive carbohydrate consumption, adequate and proper supplementation, avoiding hydrogenated and rancid fats, and consuming quality nutrient dense foods that are not genetically modified.

After 14 years of clinical practice, I have come to several conclusions. The first, and most obvious one to me, is that there is no one answer that fits everyone. You have to take people where they are as it relates to their willingness to learn and then their willingness or ability to change their lifestyle and bad habits based on their new knowledge. The second conclusion is that not everyone can afford to eat organically and purchase quality supplements or expensive water filtration systems. Thirdly, some people do not have the support and understanding of their families or peers. Lastly, biochemical individuality created by expression of genetics in response to the stimulus of our lifestyle choices, makes everyone unique.

These factors really complicate things, but must be considered. I have had to learn that health is not always the top priority for some people, and that I could not put my priorities or values onto my patients. I watched as some of these people developed the health problems I warned them about. It took developing major health challenges to change their priorities. I have also had the misfortune of seeing some of these people that I care so much about die.

I have an arsenal of comments that I make to patients to overcome various obstacles they present to me, most of the obstacles are financial. I often say, *"quality vitamins, organic foods, and pure water are a lot less expensive than visits to three or four specialists, chemotherapy, knee replacements or a heart bypass!"* Or, *"you can afford two packs of cigarettes, three soft drinks, two candy bars, and a junk food lunch every day, and a new car, but you can't afford $2.00 a day in quality* *supplements"*? Some folks get offended, but some take it to heart and move toward making better choices. It is my goal that everyone who comes to me for help, gets well and ultimately healthy in the long run. It has taken many years to know that I cannot possibly pull every one of them across the finish line. There has to be some individual accountability on the patient's part.

We started to offer free health lectures at my clinic on Monday nights. Some nights ten or more people would show up, other nights, one or two and some nights, no one would come. We couldn't even give away free health advice! It took me a while to know that people needed to have some "skin in the game" so to speak. Now there is a fee for my classes and attendance is almost perfect. It is a strange phenomenon, but people just do not want to be told what to do if they are not ready for the changes. Just because the teacher is ready doesn't mean the student will appear. All of the people in my classes now have some health problem they want to resolve. They have "skin in the game".

I usually start my first lecture by saying: *"We are born these perfect little beings. We don't care if we are a Democrat or a Republican, we don't know about hatred or racism. We are basically happy, as long as we are fed and our diapers are dry and we have adequate love. We spend 40 or 50 years messing all that up and the rest of our lives trying to get it back."* Most people who read books like this one are over forty and are in generally poor health; they are looking for another way. It usually takes that long for our unhealthy habits to catch up with us.

I have written many "guides" to attempt to explain my plan for people, most patients took them home and never read them. I have given countless hours of advice that was never taken. After giving this much thought, I felt it would be best to write a book and make it available to people who were ready for a change of course. I am glad you are at the point in your life where you know you are ready to make that change.

One of my favorite things to say to people is, *"If you don't change the things you are doing, you will keep getting the things you have."*

"If you don't change the things you are doing, you will keep getting the things you have."

Much like the concept of the food pyramid, I have been working on a "Health Pyramid". My Health Pyramid is divided into six sections which can provide a good overview of where your current health situation came from and potentially where it is going. Your health is largely under your control.

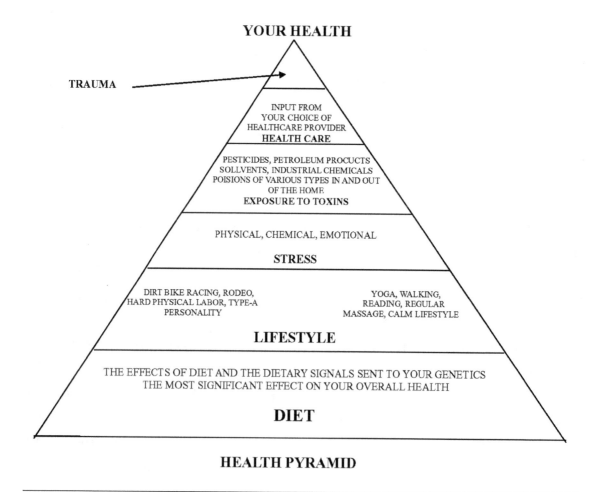

HEALTH PYRAMID

1. Diet

By far the most important factor influencing your health is your diet and the effect of that diet on your genetics. Barry Sears, the author of *The Zone Diet* said it best when he stated: *"Food is the most powerful drug you will ever encounter".* [19] Foods impact our human software that we call our genes. If you eat foods that are devoid of nutrition, no matter the amount of calories, your body will perceive that as starvation. The starvation signal is strong and suggests a threat to survival. This threat will be met with a never ending need to eat until this basic survival need is met. This is what most Americans do, send the bad messages to their genes via foods; as a result they are always looking for and thinking about foods. The human body is an incredible thing. If you take good care of it and feed it quality nutrient dense foods that send correct signals to your genes, you will have good health providing nothing traumatic happens to you.

Far too many diseases in our culture are blamed on genetics. Your genetics may be fine, it is the messages sent to your genes that are most likely to blame for diseases. Just because you have a gene for some disease does not mean it has to express itself. Genetic expression is influenced largely by lifestyle choices and diet. The following excerpt is from the book, *Rare Earths Forbidden Cures* -

> It has been clearly demonstrated in the laboratory animal, pet animal and agriculture that 98% of all birth defects are not "genetic" in nature, but in fact are the nutritional deficiencies of the egg, embryo and fetus and can be prevented by preconception nutrition. Working with these facts instead of denying them, in the animal industry has all but eliminated tragic and expensive birth defects (there are no insurance plans private or government that would cover the economic loss of a birth defect in livestock) by supplying high quality preconception and gestational nutrition to breeding animals. [20]

Most everyone has heard the phrase from your favorite computer geek, *"Garbage in, garbage out".* This is also true when it comes to the human body. If you put kerosene in a race car, it will run. It will spit and sputter and smoke, but it will run, however, it will not run very fast and will not run for long. Your body is the same way. If you continually feed it junk foods, soft drinks, excessive sugars, rancid fats and oils, poisonous food additives, sweeteners and preservatives, you will get the "garbage out" effect. The garbage out is sickness and disease. Garbage goes into the landfill. Is your body becoming a landfill?

2. Lifestyle

Lifestyle has a great effect on your overall health. If you chose to be a smoker, you can expect the fringe benefits of smoking to catch up with you sooner or later. The same is true if you use recreational drugs or alcohol. If you would rather depend on prescription drugs instead of making the necessary changes to improve your health without drugs, that too eventually comes with consequences. If you jump out of airplanes and bungee off of bridges, obviously this could have severe consequences. The point here is that you have control over your choice of lifestyle

3. Stress

I educate patients about three kinds of stress, physical, chemical, and emotional. These types of stress can have a profound effect on your overall health. If you are a daredevil, thrill seeker, if you have been injured, or if you are a workaholic, these are examples of physical stress. Chemical stress will occur if you are exposed to chemicals over prolonged periods, either at work or because you live on junk foods and have a toxic house hold. Some examples of emotional stress are road rage, depression, anxiety, type-A personality, and so on. All of these things have a long lasting influence on your overall health.

4. Exposure to Toxins

Exposure to toxins, known and unknown is common and unavoidable in America today. Our food supply, our cleaning products, our body care products, drinking water, and the air we breathe are laced with more and more chemicals and toxins every year. Some people are better able to detoxify these chemicals from their bodies than others and this certainly contributes to overall health. Infants in particular do not yet have the ability to detoxify some potential poisons. They are more vulnerable to toxins in the environment. (21)

5. Health Care

The types of health care providers and the advice they give also have an effect on your overall health. If your providers are well schooled in what creates health, you will be healthier. If you choose providers that just want to treat sickness and prescribe medications all the time, you and your doctors will create a drug dependency mentality that will never allow you to be healthy. An Ayurevedic proverb says, *"When diet is wrong, medicine is of no use. When diet is correct, medicine is of no need."*

6. Trauma

Severe trauma or permanent injuries, such as those caused by motor vehicle accidents or falls, obviously effect health and quality of life at any age. As we age we are more prone to injuries from falls, largely in part to being over medicated. (22)

A lot of people experience trauma because they are not paying attention or they are not as alert as they could be if they were healthier. If we look at it truthfully, most of the accidental traumas in our lives could have been prevented had we been paying better attention to what we were doing at the time. Recently, I saw a You Tube video of a woman who was walking through a mall while texting and fell into a small water pond. I hear of people being seriously injured because they text while they drive. I know of several people who have been seriously injured or killed while driving and texting. Traumas can have severe life altering consequences.

I am not a scientist, or a physicist, or a statistician. I am a practitioner of health. In the following chapters you will not find a lot of fancy medical terms or complicated language including long complicated words for human biochemistries or body parts. Instead, I want the information to be easily digested regardless of your current understanding of the subject material. My goal is to point out some of the simple things that you can do to influence your health in the least expensive way possible. No one could provide all the information everyone needs for everything in one book. It is also my goal to give you a viewpoint that is not always in line with the "status quo" and to give you a basic starting point to begin your quest for health. You need another point of view or another angle so that you may look at your health from a different perspective.

If you have a serious disease, or if you take a lot of prescription medications, you must consult with your primary physician about any major change in your lifestyle, or intent to discontinue taking medications. To just stop taking medications can have very harmful or potentially fatal results.

It's important to note here that there are hundreds of conflicting opinions on what is required to be healthy. It's my intention to redirect your focus. It is difficult to balance opinions on fats vs. non-fat, low carbs vs. carb loading or no carbs, vegetarian vs. non vegetarian, acid vs. alkaline diets, blood types, TV weight loss meals vs. home cooked meals, etc. The confusion presented by all of these conflicting views are hard to overcome for some people, but you have to start somewhere. If you truly have the desire to be healthy, you will find your own center as far as these issues are concerned. You must search for health or you will never find it.

You must search for health or you will never find it.

What most Americans don't know is that we are all being exposed to thousands of chemicals every day. The REGENESIS program just scratches the surface on this subject. The following pages will help make you aware of the chemicals in our foods, our home cleaning products, and especially our body care products, including cosmetics. These chemicals combined with daily stress and poor diet place an incredible toxic load on our bodies. It is impossible to be totally healthy unless you consider many things, not just your diet. If you embark on a sales career and buy a suit and a nice brief case, but never make the first call, you cannot succeed as a salesman. Put your knowledge to work!

One thing you must keep in mind is that the REGENESIS program is not a diet per se, of course there is a dietary component, but there is so much more to consider. The program is designed to decrease your "toxic burden", improve your nutrient stores via proper supplementation, and to improve and maintain your health through dietary changes. I also stress the importance of taking care of your spine and physical body using chiropractic care and other manual therapies. The program is to give you a good initial start. It is up to you to develop more knowledge through reading quality health books and articles. Reading and understanding are just one part. You must implement what you have learned into your daily routine.

Along the way, I will give many suggestions for reading material in the form of books, websites, and articles for you to research and read on your own. Remember individual accountability? You must work at being healthy. You may not agree with what you read here, that's okay. However you feel, you have to become engaged. So, having been healthy at one time in your life, you must remember how it felt. It is my hope that the information in the following chapters, will result in at least a partial or a full recovery of your health.

It is my absolute intention in the pages that follow to give you a pathway towards recovering your health. This topic is so broad and varied that it would be virtually impossible to give you everything you need in one book. Therefore, I will be giving you sources to read if you would like to further your understanding of health and wellness concepts.

I have read many books, listened to countless lectures, and helped my own patients recover their health through clinical practice. It must be understood that this book is an introduction and that each chapter could be a book in itself. I hope that once you come to realize that you can recapture your health, or at least make significant improvements, you will become thirsty for more knowledge. Give up some of your idle time in front of your televisions, put down the romance novels, and get engaged!

When I was young, my mother would point and shake her finger at me when she felt that I was not listening or not paying attention to her. There will be times in this book when it will seem like I am shaking my finger at you, I am. If you are not paying attention to what is going on around you, there are severe consequences. My mother shook her finger at me because she wanted the best for me, just as I want the best for you.

Merriam-Webster defines "*Genesis*" as: *the origin or coming into being of something*. "*Re*" is defined as: *with regard to*. The combination of these words creates REGENESIS. I chose this title as I want you to experience a coming into being healthy, a rebirth of your health. There exists in everyone, regardless of your age or your current health, a spark, a desire, and a willingness to be healthy (the scientific term for this is *homeostasis*). I hope that I can ignite a spark within you to do something different and regain your good health. I want you to experience what I call a REGENESIS!

2 | Water

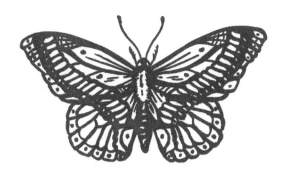

*"Water is life's matter and matrix, mother and medium.
There is no life without water."*
Albert Szent -Gyorgyi

WHEN IT COMES to reversing bad health, the first place to start is with proper hydration. This simple concept can make profound changes in your health. Depending on which source you read, your body is approximately 60% to 70% water. It seems then that it would be very important to stay hydrated and to do so with quality water. Generally speaking, most of my new patients are very poorly hydrated. We consume far too many beverages that contain water, but are not water. This will be the first challenge for most folks who are in poor health. We are a nation that consumes too many soft drinks, excessive coffee, tea and not enough pure water. It needs mentioning that the human body can survive for weeks without food, but only days without water. Quality water and proper hydration are two of the essential components required for good health.

We consume far too many things that contain water, but are not water.

Some of the physiological functions that are performed by water include: regulating body temperature, excretion, and providing a medium for all of the body's cellular elements to "float" in for circulation. Water is required for digestion and for many water dependent chemical reactions. There are many other functions of the body that require water.

The body offers many warnings when you are sub-clinically dehydrated. These symptoms are common and are often overlooked by today's healthcare practitioners. Some examples are: headaches, dry mouth, fatigue, skin problems, hypertension, asthma, poor colon health (including constipation), insomnia, arthritis, and fibromyalgia. Let's look a little closer at headaches and arthritis.

Headaches are one of the most common problems experienced by Americans, they account for a large number of visits to doctors every day. Headaches vary in many different ways from just ordinary stress type headaches, to debilitating cluster and migraine type headaches. If you have ever suffered from bad headaches, it is no wonder that you would seek some sort of intervention for them. That intervention is usually in the form of some kind of medication to make the symptom go away, and the true source of the problem is never found. Headaches can be very complicated and the sources can be many. One of the most commonly missed causes is chronic dehydration. I am talking here about sub-clinical dehydration, not like the kind of dehydration seen when someone has been throwing up for days with the flu or some other illness.

In order to understand this, you need to know that there is a rationing protocol inherent in the human body. When it comes to water, there is a kind of drought management system, a rationing system that is very important to your survival. By far, the most important need for water is for brain function. The brain is approximately 2.5 percent of the body's weight, but consumes up to 22 percent of your body energy.[1] This highly metabolic process requires a lot of water.[2] Your brain like a computer hard drive, it runs everything and it gets what it needs.

How much water do you drink? That is the first question I ask a headache patient in my office. Most of them are really dehydrated. Without proper brain function, you cannot be healthy. If the brain is not getting enough hydration, headaches are one of the results, and if the brain is not being properly hydrated, nothing else is either because the brain is number one on the priority list.

Another source of headaches, often combined with dehydration, is inflammation caused by our poor food supply and over use of wheat and wheat glutens. Wheat, glutens, and inflammation are discussed many times in the following pages.

Blood is a vital body fluid, and because of this, it also gets what it needs. How about bones, muscles, and other organs? During the fight or flight response, blood flow to the digestive organs is significantly decreased and the blood to the muscle and skeletal systems is increased. This is just one example of how your body adapts for survival.

Cartilage will suffer if you are not hydrated properly. If the dehydration continues and becomes chronic, arthritis starts to form along with degenerative joint disease. The point of this is that if you are very poorly hydrated, your brain, along with other body organs, will not function at 100%. Headaches and arthritis are potentially a by-product of this survival based water rationing system. If you suffer from headaches, most likely you will have other health issues related to dehydration as well.

This very complicated mechanism is part of the fight or flight response. I studied this briefly in my physiology classes in graduate school. However, it really became important to me after reading the book *Your Body's Many Cries for Water,* written by an Iranian doctor named F. Batmanghelidj, MD. From his book, Dr. Batmanghelidj explains:

> This complex multi-level water rationing and distribution process remains in operation until the body receives *unmistakable* signals that it has gained access to adequate water supply. Since *every function*

of the body is monitored and pegged to the flow of water, "water management" is the only way of making sure that adequate amounts of water and its transported nutrients first reach the more vital organs that will have to confront and deal with any new "stress". This mechanism became more and more established for survival against natural enemies and predators. (3)

This most informative little book is high on my suggested reading list. It can be life changing if you truly understand the hydration problem. The information in Dr. Batmanghelidj's book has helped me to assist a lot of patients that suffer from the problems associated with dehydration. Consuming quality water is a lot less expensive than multiple doctor visits and very expensive migraine medications.

Headaches are one of the major causes of lost work time and they certainly have a significant impact on a person's quality of life. For headache sufferers, just drinking an adequate amount of water every day and eliminating man made beverages would be an easy, inexpensive experiment to conduct.

Often times a dehydrated patient will complain about some kind of back or joint pain and will tell me that they were diagnosed with osteo-arthritis by their doctor. Many times the doctors will make these diagnoses without taking X-rays. I had a patient tell me she had scoliosis that had been diagnosed twelve years prior by a nurse at a high school screening. I took X-rays of her and her spine was totally straight. She cried after seeing the X-rays of her normal spine. After we made her give up soft drinks in exchange for water and corrected her spinal function with a couple of gentle chiropractic adjustments, she was more like that teenager that had been given an incorrect diagnosis so many years ago. She carried the thought of some terrible spinal affliction around with her for almost twelve years! Improper and incorrect diagnoses are common when it comes to arthritis and musculo-skeletal problems.

These osteoarthritis patients usually take over the counter or prescription medications like ibuprofen, Celebrex or other medications to relieve arthritis pain. I always ask my patients how much water they drink. Most of the people I see don't come anywhere close to their minimum water needs. Most of them drink coffee, tea, sports drinks, energy drinks, soft drinks, and maybe one small glass of water every day. They slowly become chronically dehydrated. They seek out care for their painful joints, and their doctor puts them on one of the popular arthritis drugs. Anyone who has ever taken any kind of narcotic or non-narcotic prescription pain relievers for any length of time knows that constipation is a very common side effect.(4) A major reason for constipation is dehydration.

Now we have a chronically dehydrated patient that is taking a drug that also contributes to dehydration. The actual cause of the problem in the joints is never addressed. The treatment increases the dehydration, causing the problem to get worse, even though the symptoms are much improved. Instead of getting better, the doctor's solution actually accelerates the damage and the patient is on the road to chronic joint destruction.

Now we have a chronically dehydrated patient that is taking a drug that also contributes to dehydration.

This happens every day in our drug based health care system. Instead of following prudent dietary advice including adequate <u>free</u> water, we add another (often very expensive) chemical to our body which adds to the dehydration, and the madness continues. The drug companies, the manufactured beverage companies, and the doctors make their money. The unknowing patient feels better initially, but the arthritis condition worsens over time, eventually leading to "upping" the medicine dosage. The unsuspecting patient inaccurately feels that he or she has been given the proper treatment for their diagnosis. I am not saying that people cannot benefit from medications, I have personally seen many patients that have been taking medications for a very long due to permanent joint destruction caused by osteoarthritis. Without exception, after taking their individual history, all of them have been shown to be chronically dehydrated. It is a rhetorical question, but I just wonder how they would have responded to prudent advice on proper hydration and mineral supplementation before their conditions got so bad?

In the above scenario, the medications most often cause some long term detrimental side effects. In some cases, this creates more doctor visits for a medicine induced problem, another prescription is written, and another drug is added to the list at the happy pharmacy. The patient has rented a room at the medical plantation. Merely increasing their water intake, making some dietary changes, decreasing their coffee, teas, and sodas, and adding proper supplementation would have resolved the initial problem, not just relieved the symptoms. These types of solutions last a lifetime if the patient is properly educated and truly understands the problem. Once people understand and follow realistic solutions, the problem can be solved permanently. One of my clients, a pharmacy tech, told me she has seen patients that are on as many as forty prescription drugs! The word *doctor* literally means teacher. What is your doctor teaching you? Permanent solutions or how to take medicines for the rest of your life?

Why do we stop drinking water in the proper amounts required to be healthy? I suspect the main reason is our obsession with sugar laden soft drinks and juices. It is also due to mineral deficiencies (in particular chromium and vanadium).[5] I have seen toddlers drinking out of bottles filled with sugary juices; red, black, green and orange colored soft drinks of all kinds, and chocolate milk. We develop tastes for these drinks at a very young age, and we lose our natural cravings for water. Other culprits are coffee and tea, various mineral waters, and now, power/energy drinks that are becoming more pervasive in the American diet. The move away from consuming adequate amounts of quality water towards the consumption of chemically laden man-made beverages has had devastating effects on overall human health. Most of the time these resulting health problems are not treated properly and the root causes, dehydration and chemical exposure from man-made beverages, continue to cause problems for the patient.

Soft drinks pose an interesting problem, other than the fact that they are not water. They can disrupt stomach function as well as increase insulin production. One of the easiest ways to improve acid reflux problems is to discontinue the use of soft drinks all together. Soft drinks are very acidic and cause an increase in stomach distention.[6] Another problem with soft drinks is that if you drink one soda a day (20 oz.), you are getting up to 70 grams of carbohydrates in the form of High Fructose Corn Syrup (HFCS)! This sweetener has an almost immediate influence on your triglyceride levels (one of the most detrimental fats on your cholesterol test). The dark colored soft drinks contain phosphorous and no calcium which contributes to bone loss over time. The more phosphorous containing sodas a person drinks the higher the risk of osteoporosis.[7] Long term corticosteroid use and lifestyle factors including diet can also contribute to developing osteoporosis [8] Women need to be especially aware of this because osteoporosis is more common in women than in men.

> I had a nineteen year old patient who told me he was drinking up to twenty four cans of Mountain Dew a day. He was over 300 lbs. He could not find a job and spent his days playing video games. He did not understand that he was addicted to sodas. As hard as I tried, I could not get through to him about all of the health problems that were in his future.

In Dr. Joel Wallach's book *Rare Earths Forbidden Cures,* he says:

> Chromium and vanadium deficiencies are manifested by an intense thirst for liquid high fructose corn syrup laden soft drinks being the usual first choice and water the last for mineral deficient humans and hunger for carbohydrates (i.e. - soft drinks, coffee and tea with added sugar, alcohol, pasta, desserts, bread, etc,).
> The "munchies", cravings for alcohol and candy cravings (especially chocolate) are sure signs of a chromium and vanadium deficiencies. (9)

These cravings are especially present in pre-teens and teenagers. Sweet cravings carry over into adulthood and are seen in diabetics in particular. Chromium and vanadium supplementation is very effective for diabetics provided an additional twenty three co-factors needed for biochemical reactions are present. The majority of these co-factors are minerals. Most people do not consume all of the necessary co-factors; therefore, it is incumbent on the diabetic patient, and everyone else for that matter, to supplement properly. Unfortunately, most doctors are completely unaware of this as they are not educated in nutritional approaches to health, so conditions like diabetes that my mother endured for years, continue to ravage our nation in lives and in cost.

Diet drinks are no better than regular soft drinks. In fact, they are worse for your health than the sugar laced sodas. Using products containing Nutra-Sweet (aspartame) makes people think that they are making a healthy choice over conventional sodas. They are mistaken. Aspartame has been the topic of much debate. I have seen local doctors and nurses in my community drinking diet drinks! We will be discussing Aspartame, other artificial sweeteners, and some common food chemicals later in the book. Eliminating soft drinks (all kinds) and replacing them with pure water almost immediately begins improving your health.

Eliminating soft drinks (all kinds) and replacing them with pure water almost immediately begins improving your health.

When I have the water consumption conversation with coffee drinkers, it is equally challenging. Once you run water through ground coffee beans, it is no longer water. Coffee tastes great, I like an occasional cup of coffee myself, however, drinking one or two pots of coffee a day thinking you are hydrating yourself is folly as coffee exerts a significant dehydrating effect [10]. Coffee does contain water, however, it also contains chemicals and natural substances that require large amounts of water for digestion which increases the work load of the kidneys due to the diuretic effects. This takes away from the natural reserves of water that your body has access to. It has been my experience that most people do not really have much "reserve" of water in their bodies. Regular tea has basically the same effect as coffee, but to a lesser degree. Some of the more subtle caffeine free herbal teas do not have the same dehydrating effect on the body. None of these beverages are a substitute for pure water.

When patients are trying to make the transition from manufactured beverages to natural water, they often complain that they don't like water and need something for flavoring. When I hear this, I know that the patient is severely dehydrated. The cravings for water are as natural as going to sleep, swallowing, and blinking your eyes. My usual answer to this problem is to use lemon or lime and a couple of drops of stevia to flavor the water. Using lemons and limes decreases your cravings for sugar. It cannot be stressed enough that one must eliminate manufactured beverages and drink water until the natural cravings for water return.

What kind of water is best? There are seemingly hundreds of different types of water available. To keep things simple in this book, I have a reasonable answer to this question.

I am a big fan of the Berkey filter. It is a stainless steel gravity filter that is very inexpensive when compared to other filters. They can be purchased for around 200 dollars. I have a link to them posted on www.regenesis4health.com. If this is a little too expensive, try one of the popular pitcher type filters. This is a reasonable start. It's important to filter out chlorine, fluoride and other harmful chemicals. Where you live and the source of your water makes a difference in the type of filter you may require. There is a wide range of prices on water filtration systems. One of my goals is to help you get started on changing your health as inexpensively as possible. If you want to invest in a water purification system that alkalizes and purifies your water (like a Kangen unit), it is certainly worthwhile to do your research and purchase one if your finances allow for it.

Our lifestyle choices, our stress, and our food choices can create an overly acidic environment in our bodies. If you follow the REGENESIS program, your overall pH will improve by proper hydration and proper food choices. When it comes to pH, it is always best if your water is on the alkaline side of the pH scale. Kits for testing pH are very inexpensive. It is eye opening to test the pH of anything you drink! Most of our manufactured beverages are extremely acidic. They are in the three to five range on the pH scale, where seven is neutral. We will be addressing body pH in chapter eleven.

If you live somewhere that utilizes a municipal water system, it will most likely use the standard types of chemicals for water purification. Chlorine and fluoride are often used depending on local water treatment guidelines. If municipal water exceeds allowable limits for bacteria or heavy metals, the municipalities are required by law to notify you of these concerns. Often times it is days or weeks before the consumers of municipal water become aware they have been drinking water with elevated levels of heavy metals. The average pH of drinking water is around seven, there are generally small variations of pH in water from different sources. Municipal water utilities are required to notify users if the pH moves too far in either direction from the neutral pH of seven. The Berkey filter removes these standard chemicals and most heavy metals. The Berkey filter is not designed to significantly impact pH. There are many systems that do this but can cost hundreds or thousands of dollars. It is like golf, you can spend as much money as you want; the decision is entirely up to you.

On the upper end of water purifiers, I am a huge proponent of the Kangen water systems. This type of water was invented in Japan in the 1950's. In Japan, the Kangen units are used in hospital settings and are considered medical modalities. These systems create clustered water that is highly absorbable and high in antioxidants. The units create varying degrees of alkaline and acid water. Alkaline water is good for changing the body's internal biological terrain to a more alkaline state. Acidic water is very useful for skin issues and general cleaning usage. Kangen units are pricey, but they can provide significant health benefits to a person with serious health challenges.

...what goes down into the ground must come up in the wells and springs.

If you drink from a well or a spring, don't be fooled into thinking that you are drinking pure water. If you live in an agricultural area, water sources can come from miles away and can contain agrichemicals, pesticides, or herbicides. It is important to understand that what goes down into the ground must come up in the wells and springs. This is very important because wells and springs, in addition to municipal water supplies, can have high concentrations of pesticides, herbicides, and heavy metals like lead.[11] It would be wise to have your water tested if you really want to know if it is pure (include a water radon test too). Most local extension agents can help you get your water tested or you may find an independent contractor who can test it for you. Living in the country or drinking chemically treated water from municipal water plants does not shield you from potential water problems.

Living in the country or drinking chemically treated water from municipal water plants does not shield you from potential water problems.

I am not a fan of distilled water as it contains no minerals and is also a powerful solvent. Reverse osmosis (RO) systems tend to acidify the water, can be expensive, and can sometimes be difficult to maintain. Bottled water warrants much discussion. I don't want to spend too much time on that, but it's important to say a few basic things here. This may help in purchasing bottled water if you don't have access to your own pure water supply.

Water companies often make bold claims when in reality their water is just charcoal filtered and often comes from a municipal water supply. Have you taken the time to compare a gallon of water purchased in 16 oz. bottles to a gallon of gas? In that form, we pay way more for water than we do for a gallon of gas. There are colored, fancy glass bottles, aluminum bottles, stainless steel bottles, plastic bottles, and sports bottles with various tops on them. Water has become quite a profitable industry, to say the least.

Plastics contain chemicals that can leach out into the water. An accumulation of these chemicals in your body can have long term health consequences. It's important to know which plastics are acceptable. If you have to buy water, glass bottles are preferable. Throw away plastic bottles are usually made of polyethylene terephthalate (PTE or PETE) and have a resin ID code of 1. High density polyethylene (HDPE) has a resin ID code of 2. Low density polyethylene (LDPE) has a resin ID code of

4. Polypropylene (PP) has a resin ID code of 5. Of all the plastics the ones with ID codes of 1, 2, 4, and 5 are considered the safest.(12) Glass bottles are always preferred and stainless steel bottles are good too. Violet colored glass water containers are optimal if you become a water bottle connoisseur. As a side note here, most bottled waters are on the acidic side of the pH scale.

An example of a typical resin ID code found on all plastic containers, in this case, resin ID code 1.

Some plastic water bottles can leach out chemicals that are known carcinogens and xenoestrogens (synthetic or natural chemicals that mimic hormones). Freezing water bottles increases the leeching effect. Plastic bottles with a resin code 7 is most highly associated with BPA.(13) Chemicals from plastic resins can have detrimental health consequences including cancer, endocrine disruption, and liver problems.(14) This is an area of research that is ongoing, so to be safe, use a glass bottle if possible.

There have been many theories as to how much water one should drink on a daily basis. This requirement depends on how big or small you are. For general starting purposes, I have adopted a simple formula in my clinic. You should consume ½ of your body weight in ounces of water per day. For example, a 100 lb. person should consume 50 oz. of water per day. A 200 lb. person would need 100 oz. per day. Once you are fully participating in the REGENESIS program, your natural thirst will be your guide for water intake.

You should consume ½ of your body weight in ounces of water per day

Club soda is acceptable. To add some flavor, use some lemon or lime along with some stevia drops and a touch of sea salt. This formula may help you to wean yourself from carbonated soft drinks.

If you have kidney or other issues related to fluid retention and are not able to process larger amounts of water, you should proceed slowly and increase your water intake gradually. If you have a serious kidney issue, you should consult with your kidney specialist. If you drink too much water, you can deplete your body of electrolytes, which can actually be fatal. It takes a lot of water in a short amount of time to do this, but it is possible.

Hydration is not merely a water deficiency problem. Supplementation with minerals is the key to proper long term hydration. Minerals affect proper and adequate fluid exchange at the cellular level. If you are losing water due to high intensity work or sports, merely drinking water will not provide adequate hydration. Mineral supplementation is discussed at length in chapter nine.

Do yourself a favor, exchange manufactured beverages for water and educate yourself on how to purify and carry your water for your daily use. You will start to see the changes in your health in just a few days. This is a crucial consideration if you are ever going to get healthy and stay healthy. Pure water is an essential component for success on the REGENESIS program!

3

Wheat
The ugly, the bad, the good.

"Be careful reading health books, you may die of a misprint."
Mark Twain

The ugly, the bad

This is one of the most important topics of the entire book! Understanding the wheat problem will be the key to your success. I wanted to start with the ugly and the bad because our obsession with wheat and wheat products is one of, if not the biggest challenges in reclaiming our health. There is a general rule of thumb when it comes to food: *Eat local grown foods in season.* If you just go by that rule, wheat would not be as much of a problem. Wheat is never in season 365 days a year. Most people consume wheat several times a day. I always get "that look" when I tell a patient to give up their wheat. This includes, pasta noodles, cereals, cakes, cookies, pancakes, gravy biscuits (a Virginia favorite), waffles, soups, and all of the seemingly thousands of things that contain wheat. I have spent so much time trying to explain why today's man-made wheat is such a problem.

Wheat is never in season 365 days a year.

Let's start with the seeds used in the wheat industry. The seeds used today are a far cry from the wheat seeds that were used in biblical times. Wheat has been hybridized, cross-bred (intentionally and unintentionally), for decades now. Hybridization keep the "bugs" off of the crop and increases yield. If the "bugs" won't eat it, we should avoid it as well. Aren't we smarter than the bugs? Today's wheat is shorter in stature, allowing the plant to yield more and it shortens the growing season. Hybridization has caused major shifts in the content and genetic make-up of wheat and the wheat proteins gluten and gliadin. (1)

There are thousands of types of wheat, but only a select few are used by today's wheat farmers. The primary wheat used by growers today is extremely hybridized *Triticum aestivum*.(2) To start with, seeds are treated with fungicides and insecticides before they are planted in order to prevent or control diseases and pests. Often times, the seeds are treated with a "cocktail" of these chemicals to control a broader spectrum of diseases and pests.(3) So even before farmers get seeds into the ground there is a problem.

As usual, these chemicals are deemed safe by the Food and Drug Association. Chemicals of all types, regardless of where they come from, increase the toxic burden that contributes to poor health. I don't care if they are approved by the FDA. The FDA approves a lot of things that were proven in the long run to be unhealthy. Remember VIOXX? Thousands of people died taking FDA approved Vioxx. Research on Vioxx revealed the potential to cause fatal heart problems, and still the drug was released to an unknowing public. (4)

Once in the ground, the wheat seeds receive more pesticides, fertilizers, and chemicals. Again this is done to increase yield. Fertilizers must be used because the soils are farmed over and over again depleting the soil of vital minerals.(5) Most plants will grow using fertilizers with only three ingredients: nitrogen, phosphorous, and potassium (N-P-K).

We humans need 60 minerals every day to be healthy. Our modern foods are not giving us anything close to the daily mineral requirements we need. We will return to minerals many times in this book as they are an essential part of the REGENESIS program.

When wheat is mass produced, it must be stored in mass as well. Storage of wheat presents its own set of problems. Insects love wheat in storage therefore, to combat this the industry uses chemical "protectants". These protectants are used around the bins and also on top of the wheat. Using some specific testing methods, if one live insect is found, the entire storage bin is fumigated to protect the wheat until it is transported.[6] More chemicals! Are you seeing a disturbing pattern here? This is all necessary to increase yield so that we can feed an ever expanding world population and America's wheat addiction.

There is another consideration that we must talk about, processing. Back in biblical times, wheat was stone ground. It was literally ground between two large stones. Stone grinding allows all of the constituents of the wheat to be present in the final product. This was, and is still the best way to process wheat, but it takes time. When processing wheat by the ton, stone grinding wheat berries takes too long. Now we get into high speed, high heat milling (this allowed us to create white flour), and this is an area that causes more problems.

The bran and the germ of the wheat are removed during the milling process, and we are left with the least nutritious part of the wheat berry, the endosperm. Most of the vitamins and minerals in the wheat are lost at this point. Quality heirloom organic whole wheat, consciously grown, is loaded with vitamins. Depending on where it is grown, it may also be rich in minerals. For the most part, we are not dealing with heirloom organic wheat we are dealing with the chemical laden hybridized variety that has been stored in bins treated with pesticides. The end product of this milling process is "refined" flour. Since most of the nutrition was discarded, bread manufacturers "enrich" their breads with synthetic vitamins. They use this as a positive selling point. Enriched whole wheat bread sounds healthy to the uneducated consumer.

There is still more "stuff" put in the bread by the manufacturers. Hydrogenated fats, conditioners, leavening agents like sodium aluminum sulfate and other ingredients are added to get the desired effect and create a loaf of bread that is appealing to the consumer. These breads will last through delivery, several days on the store shelf, and several days in your homes, all of which increases profitability. In the end, the bread product you get is a massively hybridized, chemical laden, highly processed, vitamin and mineral depleted frankenfood.

Variations of this processing will create pasta noodles, cereals, gluten products, fillers used in other food products, and animal foods. They do not throw anything away. These foods end up in our homes and in our bellies, now the problem with wheat gets personal. Highly processed wheat contributes largely to our civilized diseases and health problems. Today's wheat is one of the most common food allergies in America because of its massive hybridization and over consumption. It is the source of Celiac disease, wheat allergies, wheat sensitivities, and nutrient malabsorption problems. Malabsorption occurs when the body can no longer absorb nutrients efficiently and is a contributing factor in many other diseases discussed in future chapters.

Today's wheat is much higher in gluten content than its biblical ancestors.

Today's wheat is much higher in gluten content than its biblical ancestors. The gluten found in wheat today is highly reactive in some people (Celiac disease), and less reactive in others. Many Americans have problems with wheat ranging from general sensitivity, allergies, Irritable Bowel Syndrome (IBS), Celiac disease, ulcerative colitis, and Crohn's disease.

This highly reactive gluten protein is consumed almost daily by most Americans. Some folks eat it multiple times a day in various forms. The United Stated Department of Agriculture (USDA) food pyramid used grains as the foundation to its daily food intake guidelines. Americans were told to stop eating saturated fats and replace the lost calories with wholesome grains, mainly wheat. Over consumption of wheat often causes an irritation in the gut, particularly in the intestines. Over time this irritation and consequent inflammation can contribute to, or cause a multitude of health problems. This includes neurological diseases[7], IBS, acid reflux, fatigue, fibromyalgia, arthritis, diabetes, obesity, insomnia, asthma, skin problems like, acne, eczema, and psoriasis.[8] It is my intention to make perfectly clear in the following lines just how insidious the damage is when one consumes today's modern hybridized and highly processed wheat.

Not only is the gluten in wheat a problem, but today's wheat, *Triticum aestivum*, is a major cause of blood sugar issues. Most people are unaware of how wheat can cause unhealthy spikes in blood sugar and consequently blood insulin levels. According to the glycemic index (a measure of the effects of different carbohydrates on blood sugar levels), 2 slices of whole wheat bread can raise your blood sugar levels as much or more than a can of soda or a Snickers bar. [9]

Both white and especially whole wheat, contributes dramatically to your overall sugar consumption. This is one of the major sources of hidden sugars that I have to teach my patients about. If you are a diabetic, you must avoid wheat. This is counter to what diabetics are taught by nutritionists at the hospital when they attend diabetic classes on how to eat. Patients are taught about the importance of grains (especially wheat) and the beneficial fiber contained in grains. These classes can cost over $2,000.00 and are covered by most insurance policies. I am still waiting for someone to explain the logic in that one.

I remember once when I was staying with my mother on one of her many protracted stays in the hospital, her hospital "nutritionist" popped in and spoke with her briefly about what she wanted her to eat as they felt she was eating too much salt (at the same time she had an IV bag full of sodium chloride going into her arm). I looked at the list of foods to eat and I was alarmed at the recommendations. I asked her if she was going to use this list, and she told me, "I'm not going to change anything. I have been eating this way all of my life. You can take that if you want it". I re-typed the information in the handout (to avoid any copyright infringement because of some art work on the original) to show you how ignorant of proper nutrition some hospital "nutritionists" are. Notice on "A Guide to Choosing Low-Sodium Foods" (see next page) that it suggests at least six servings a day of "breads, pasta, cereals, baked goods and rice". I absolutely will not allow doughnuts, pancakes, waffles, shredded wheat and the like on the REGENESIS plan, especially for a diabetic. These recommendations are what keep people in the diabetic state! Perhaps that is the goal? Diabetics are worth a lot to the health care system in medicines, doctor visits, amputations, peripheral neuropathies, hospital stays, insulin, blood sugar testing equipment, bed sore management, oxygen tanks, kidney specialists, and so on. From a purely business perspective, why would you ever want to get a cash cow like that well?

Irritation / Inflammation

Once the wheat has made its way to your house in various forms, it is usually over consumed for a variety of reasons. It is inexpensive, convenient and delicious. The Chinese have a saying, "nothing to excess" for they believe that out of excess comes deficiency. If there is anything in the typical American diet that is done to excess, it's wheat. If you consume a product that is by its very nature an irritant, (gluten looks like a porcupine under a microscope), it will lead to inflammation. If you have Celiac disease, eating wheat is like eating a poison ivy salad.

A Guide to Choosing Low Sodium Foods

Food Group	Low Sodium Foods	High Sodium Foods
*Breads *Cereals *Pasta *Rice *Baked Goods *At least 6 servings Per day	**Unsalted Grain Products:** -Hot Cereals -Macaroni and other plain noodles -Shredded Wheat -Corn Tortillas -Unsalted popcorn -Low Sodium breads and crackers -Rice **Use these products in moderation** -Breads and rolls -Pies and Pastries -Doughnuts -Pancakes and Waffles -Dry Cereals	**Highly Salted Grain** -Instant hot cereals -Pretzels -Salted Chips/crackers -Popcorn (salted) -Commercial rice or Pasta dishes

Nutritional information given to my severely diabetic mother in the hospital

It is this inflammatory process that starts a host of events depending on how sensitive or reactive your system is to wheat. If you consume wheat several times a day, the gut never gets a break from it. This inflammation proceeds insidiously every day for years. Once the intestines are irritated, they no longer absorb nutrients properly, this is a common cause of the malabsorption issues that create a host of health problems. An interesting side note here is that this inflammation causes our bodies to produce cholesterol, not quality dietary fat as we have been led to believe.[10] We will spend more time on cholesterol later.

Once the intestines are irritated, they no longer absorb nutrients properly

LEAKY GUT SYNDROME
(aka Increased Intestinal Permeability)

Let's do a little anatomy here. In your small intestine on the inner wall is a structure called the brush border, it is comprised of finger like projections called villi. These villi project inwards to give more surface area to absorb digested food particles. If these projections were flattened out totally like pizza dough, it would create a surface area larger than a tennis court. All along the surface of the brush border lining is an immunoglobulin called secretory IgA (a protein produced by the immune system) and trillions of bacteria and yeast called the gut flora. Secretory IgA is very important in preventing infections and can be severely depleted in people with leaky gut syndrome. This alone can severely limit the immune function that is intrinsic to the intestines. These trillions of bacteria (gut flora, aka probiotics) are supposed to be there along with yeast. They are "good bacteria" and have a very specific function. As long as the yeast and bacteria are in balance, all is well.

There are many types of gut bacteria along with the yeast. They have a symbiotic relationship with each other, meaning they all rely on each other for survival. The purpose of this gut flora is to break down foods into very small particles, so that they can be absorbed into the bloodstream and carried off to the liver to be processed. The gut flora also synthesizes vitamins and amino acids. Once foods processed in the intestine pass through the liver, the body takes these nutrients and uses them for thousands of functions in order to fuel and maintain our bodies.

The gut is a crucial player in overall immune function. In the mucus producing superficial layers of the gut lining, we find the gut associated lymphoid tissue (GALT), consisting of Peyer's patches, various lymphocyte (a type of white blood cell) producing cells, and microfold cells. These cells located at the superficial layer of the gut lining manufacture the previously mentioned secretory IgA, and other important immune system secretions. The GALT cells are one of the body's first lines of defense as it relates to immune function. If this gut lining is compromised, it can have a profound effect on overall immunity. If the gut lining is unhealthy, the individual will be more susceptible to infections. If you are the type of person that stays tired and or sick all of the time, it is very possible that you have a problem in your gut.

If you are the type of person that stays tired and or sick all of the time, it is very possible that you have a problem with your gut.

Under normal circumstances, small particles of digested food pass thru small channels or junctions called *desmosomes* that exists between the cells of the small intestines. When the small intestine has all the co-factors, enzymes, and vitamins needed and is free of irritation, it will function properly. When a constant irritation of the small intestine occurs, this proper gut function is interrupted and we can develop a condition called "leaky gut syndrome". In order for the body to combat the irritation and subsequent infections that develop in a poorly functioning intestine, these small channels between the cells have to get larger. This is needed to allow large white blood cells to pass from the blood supply into the lining of the small intestine. When these small channels open up, it causes an increase in the intestinal permeability allowing food particles that are larger than normal to be absorbed in reverse into the bloodstream. The gut leaks these larger particles like a sieve that is too big. (11)

Once in the bloodstream, the body does not recognize these abnormally large food particles. The immune system thinks these particles are foreign or pathogenic and attacks them for removal. This is an immune response to food. Now the patient has circulating antibodies to foods, this is one of the ways we develop a food sensitivity or a food allergy. The abnormal immune response to food caused by leaky gut syndrome requires a lot of energy. This explains why people with leaky gut syndrome always experience some degree of fatigue. (12)

There is a great test that measures your immune response to these food particles called the ALCAT test. It is a live blood analysis and is not widely used in the medical field yet. I have had very good results when patients put the ALCAT information to use. According to ALCAT researchers, the test is 83% accurate. (13) This is very high as far as measuring food allergy or sensitivity. Testing for IgG-4 delayed food allergies is another useful blood test.

The problem does not end there. Often times this process is caused by chronic stress, alcohol, commercially grown meats, and chlorinated water (chlorine kills the gut bacteria). Sometimes the person is given antibiotics and/or anti-inflammatory drugs to treat their small intestine problem. Their doctor may perceive the patient's complaints as an illness that requires medicines, the plot thickens. Once the good bacteria are killed off in significant numbers, the yeast that lives there, takes over. This is why a lot of women get a yeast infection while taking antibiotics. Men develop yeast problems as well; they are just not as keenly aware of it. In men, it will most often present as a skin rash, itching or both.

Systemic yeast problems create a long list of symptoms. "Candidiasis" and "moniliasis" are other terms used for severe yeast problems.

The intestinal flora is now seriously out of balance. This is a condition called "dysbiosis". Now the patient is almost always sick because their immunity is severely compromised by the compounding problems. They get more antibiotics and develop yeast infections, parasites, pain, fatigue, gas and bloating. At this point, patients are usually prescribed medicines like Nystatin that kill yeast overgrowth. Now we have a very serious long term health problem. It is at this time that the intestinal balance must be restored to normal. This rarely happens. To correct dysbiosis, the problems that created it must be resolved. Most MD's and nutritionists are not trained to even recognize, much less repair the problem. I had a patient that told her doctor she had a "leaky gut". He laughed and said he had never heard of such a ridiculous thing. There are medical tests for increased intestinal permeability, aka "leaky gut syndrome". If left undiagnosed, the patient's gut problem is never resolved and they seem to feel bad all the time. These people slowly begin to develop multiple health problems and a general decline in overall health and vitality.

the patient's gut problem is never resolved and they seem to feel bad all the time.

Years into this process the malabsorption is well established and the diseases start to show up. These can include chronic fatigue, allergies, hypertension, lupus, MS, arthritis, constipation and or diarrhea, neurological diseases, depression, irritable bowel syndrome, ulcerative colitis, skin problems, asthma, fibromyalgia, food cravings, obesity, diabetes, insomnia, Celiac disease, Crohn's disease, and cancer in the worst of cases. All too often, these symptoms and diseases are treated with more medicines or surgeries while the underlying cause remains undiagnosed and improperly treated. It's not uncommon for a Celiac disease patient to go more than ten years without a proper diagnosis. Dr. Joseph Murray M.D. the director of the Mayo Clinic's Celiac Clinic says:

> *Besides the risk of osteoporosis, iron deficiency anemia and other direct consequences of malabsorption, Celiac's disease is associated with excess mortality due to malignancy, particularly non-Hodgkin's Lymphoma. Mortality increases when diagnosis is delayed more than 10 years.... While Celiac disease in its' classic form, severe malabsorption, is seen by gastroenterologists, most patients won't present with this but with a wide diversity of less well defined conditions.* (14)

This is why the disease is often misdiagnosed or missed altogether. It's difficult for a doctor to catch this with just three to five minutes of face to face time with patients. Some medical doctors will see 50 or more patients a day. Unfortunately, this is how modern medicine is carried out on a day to day basis in this country. This system does not allow very much one on one time for the doctor and the patient.

Research suggests that today's highly hybridized, cross pollenated, toxic, wheat has led to increased intestinal problems including: wheat allergy, irritable bowel syndrome, Celiac disease and colon cancer.(15) This wheat problem can begin in infancy and can be passed through the placenta from the mother to her unborn child. All too often infants are fed wheat way too early for their intestinal tracts to process it.

From our earlier discussion we know how toxic and irritating our wheat supply is. Symptoms of wheat allergy or Celiac disease can be seen in infants. They include:

SKIN REACTIONS: Hives, red bumps, eczema

BREATHING EFFECTS: wheezing, asthma, and in severe cases anaphylaxis

DIGESTIVE EFFECTS: gas, bloating, nausea, diarrhea and diaper rash, excessive crying due to intestinal pain. In severe cases bloody stool.

PSYCHOLOGICAL EFFECTS: irritability, crankiness, headaches, hyperactivity, tantrums, and anxiety. [16]

Celiac disease is very easy to miss; even the specialists miss it sometimes. If it can be overlooked in its most severe form in a small child, imagine how easy it is to miss in an adult with several seemingly unconnected symptoms. If you currently have at least three or more chronic health problems, it is very possible that you have a malabsorption problem caused by a wheat sensitivity or even Celiac disease. Have yourself tested. There is a blood test that measures circulating antibodies to wheat and is fairly accurate. The ALCAT test is another one you could do. If you suspect that you are wheat sensitive, you could just eliminate it from your diet all together for several months. I would bet that most of you would feel much better in just a few days or weeks by doing this simple experiment. This method does not cost anything.

There is mounting evidence that wheat sensitivities can contribute to peripheral neuropathy, rheumatoid arthritis, lymphoma, and pancreatic cancer [17, 18, 19]. Wheat is one of the foods at the foundation of the familiar food pyramid established in 1992 by the USDA which suggests 6 to 11 servings of grains daily. The food pyramid has been replaced by the supposedly more reasonable Harvard "food plate", which is still basically the old "prudent diet" that demonizes saturated fats, promotes whole grains, and man-made polyunsaturated fats. Since the implementation of the USDA food pyramid, diabetes and obesity have skyrocketed in

America.(20) So this food that is so potentially dangerous to so many has been endorsed by the government (that subsidizes grain production), for over two decades.

There is a sophisticated brain/gut connection that is way beyond the scope of this book. In order to understand this relationship more, again I would suggest the book *Gut and Psychology Syndrome*, written by a Russian MD, Dr. Natasha Campbell-McBride.(21) She does a great job of explaining how the gut affects the psychology of both children and adults. The connection to the gut and depression, Tourette's syndrome, ADHD, anxiety, schizophrenia, bi-polar disorder, and autism is emerging. This correlates with inflammation of the brain caused by gluten proteins and the interruption of the production of serotonin. This interruption of serotonin production can occur in people with wheat sensitivities or Celiac disease and/or from the serotonin re-uptake inhibitors (SSRI) drugs like Prozac, Zoloft, and others. It has been suggested that wheat sensitivities and Celiac disease cause an alteration in the natural production and utilization of serotonin. (22) SSRI's are highly profitable drugs and have made the manufacturers billions of dollars. Why is the public so misinformed about this? Another great book about this is *Grain Brain* by Dr. David Perlmutter. (23)

This is a good place to splice in some discussion on genetic modification. Genetically modified corn, soy, tomatoes, cottonseed, canola oils, beet sugars, yellow squash, and many other foods are prevalent in our food supply. One food in particular, corn and anything made from GMO corn (like corn chips, corn meal etc.), create a toxin called Bt-toxin. The reason I want to mention this here is because Bt-toxin is designed to kill the bugs that eat corn crops by punching holes in their digestive tracts. Studies show that this toxin also punches holes in human cells too. It has been suggested that this is one of the reasons for the increase in five gluten related digestive conditions. They are (1) Increased intestinal permeability, (2) imbalanced gut flora, (3) immune activation and allergies, (4) impaired digestion, (5) damage to the intestinal wall.[24] Again "It's not nice to fool Mother Nature".

I hope I have provided some insight as to why wheat is not the healthy food it is portrayed to be. I feel that it is possibly the root cause of a lot of things that we seek medical care for, especially the chronic health conditions. It was not always that way, so I would like to address the good parts of wheat.

The Good

I know people that have been smoking for fifty years and are healthy as a mule. There are some people who can consume wheat with no problems, but I think this warrants some significant explanation. It was during the time when mankind was moving from a lifestyle of hunter gatherer to one of cultivation and domestication that grains and dairy were introduced into the diets of our ancient ancestors. The gluten proteins found in wheat, corn, rye, and barley are very hard for humans to digest. There are ancient human bloodlines that tend to do better with consuming grains than others. Asians are a good example as they have been using grains (mainly rice) as a food staple for thousands of years. Genetically they have larger endocrine glands that allow for more complete digestion of grains when compared to people of western societies.

There are some things that can make grains, especially wheat, more digestible. Phytates are salts or esters of phytic acid that occur in grains and are insoluble. They require other vitamins and minerals to be processed by the body and, therefore, are called anti-nutrients which deplete the body of nutrients. Soaking grains in water breaks down phytates, and makes grains more digestible. Examples of this are sourdough bread or sprouted breads. As for dairy, fermenting and culturing milk proteins also makes them more digestible. We will touch on dairy in a future chapter.

Even if you think that you are okay with wheat, it is not allowed on the REGENESIS program.

Discussing wheat must naturally start with one of the organic grains used in biblical times. There are approximately 30,000 kinds of wheat in the world. Historians believe that the Einkorn type of wheat was used most during biblical times. Emmer wheat is another ancient type of wheat. Some sources date these species back as far as 10,000 to 15,000 BC.[25] Einkorn has only a fraction of the gluten found in modern day wheat. It is highly nutritious, but it is hard to find. It has a very different taste than today's wheat. Einkorn wheat is not as co-operative as modern wheat in that the dough made from it does not mold well. It would be almost impossible to make a donut or calzone out of Einkorn wheat.[26]

There are several good sources of Einkorn wheat online. Even Einkorn wheat is something that should not be consumed very often, remember, nothing to excess. I would suggest using even this type of wheat sparingly. For purposes of reclaiming your health, I would allow you try this kind of wheat only after you have reached a "healthy" state. Totally wheat free is still my ultimate goal for people on the REGENESIS program.

I can't emphasize enough that people with Celiac or Crohn's disease must avoid these gluten containing grains even if they are sprouted or soaked. If you are diabetic or your purpose is weight loss, I suggest that you do a completely grain free diet. If you have health problems or you are just unhealthy in general, I also suggest a grain free lifestyle. Remember there are several problems with processed wheat: chemicals, pesticides, fungicides, hybridization (by man not by nature), processing, extrusion (using high heat to turn wheat into little 0's and puffs, etc.), food additives, high carbohydrate and gluten content, and for sure excess consumption.

To clear up some confusion, processed quick oats are not allowed on the REGENESIS program because they do contain significant carbohydrates and some gluten. The gluten is not in the grain itself but is in the final product as these grains are usually processed in the same factories that process wheat products. This allows for a kind of cross contamination to occur. If the oats say "gluten free" on the packaging, this means that they were processed in a factory that only processes oats. Gluten free steel cut oats are allowed, but only in small servings as they do tend to cause an increased insulin response. If you are diabetic or want to lose weight, even steel cut organic oats are not allowed.

Early on in this chapter, I documented some information from the book *Wheat Belly,* by Dr. William Davis. Dr. Davis a preventative cardiologist in Michigan. His book is one of the most informative hard hitting books on wheat I have ever read. If you have any doubts about why wheat is a "bad food", and if you still think that today's wheat is a healthy food, *Wheat Belly* will remove any doubts you have. *Wheat Belly* and *Grain Brain* by Dr. David Perlmutter are very high on my must read list. If you don't understand the problem with modern wheat after reading these two books, you are unreachable.

One thing that really stands out to me while I was researching information on this chapter, is the vast amount of research that has been done on how harmful modern wheat and wheat glutens are on human health and how little our doctors and health community really know about it. I know this because they continue to promote it and advise people on how important wheat and grains are. Patients have brought me various hand-outs they get from their doctors regarding diet. It is the prudent diet in every case, high in grains and still recommending PUFA's (man-made polyunsaturated fatty acids) and very limited or no quality saturated fats. Get use to me slamming the "prudent diet", it is tied to my whipping post.

In summary, you should be drinking good water instead of man-made beverages, and you should be removing all of the wheat products from your diet. Your journey towards better health has begun.

4

Sugars (Carbohydrates)

"We want our health and eat our sugarcake too."
William Dufty (Sugar Blues)

I GET MORE questions and have more arguments over sugar than anything. Americans are addicted to sugar. Depending on which estimate you read, Americans consume an average of 157 lbs. of sugar per person, per year.(1) Around 1900, the average sugar consumption was between one and five pounds per person per year. How did that happen? Go to any convenience store about 30 minutes before the local school system starts in the morning. You will see high school aged kids and the general public, stocking up on their daily sugary soft drinks, energy drinks, candy bars, coffee, cappuccinos, and sugary wheat snack favorites like donuts. Throw in a couple packs of dipping snuff or cigarettes for some of them and you have a day full of disease causing fun. It is truly an eye opening experience.

Other than gold, silver, and now oil, sugar has contributed to the demise of several great empires and great armies, from the Arab conquerors to the Christian crusaders. It was a major contributor to the burgeoning slave trade initiated in the 1400's.(2) Now it has contributed greatly to the destruction of our great nation's health. I was watching a talk show on TV and heard one of the pundits say something that struck me right between the eyes. I am paraphrasing, but he said something to the effect that America could not fight another world war because of the health of our young adults. I am certainly no fan of world wars, but if one takes a truly objective look around, he is probably right. As a nation we are nowhere near as physically fit and healthy as we were back in the early 1900's.

There are many forms of sugar.

There are many forms of sugar. For the purposes of this book, the words sugar and carbohydrates mean the same thing. Carbohydrate is a term used to describe sugars either single molecules or molecules hooked together in a chain. I divide sugars into two main groups, the simple carbohydrates (sugars), and the complex carbohydrates (sugars).

The simple sugars are monosaccharides containing one sugar molecule, and disaccharides that contain two sugar molecules. The complex sugars, oligosaccharides, contain three or more (potentially thousands of molecules). The simple sugars are absorbed into the bloodstream very quickly as they have only one or two molecules. These types of sugars are very common in our fast foods and our national food supply. White table sugar and high fructose corn syrups are simple sugars; fruits also contain a simple sugar, fructose. A word about fruits here; fruits contain varying amounts of fiber which offsets the speed and degree of absorption of fructose. Since the REGENESIS program is about lowering blood sugars and therefore the insulin response, I tend not to allow high sugar low fiber fruits on the plan.

It's important to know all of the sources of sugars, but there are particular sources of sugar that must be understood, processed wheat products, high fructose corn syrup, and processed white sugar. There has been considerable debate over the years as to whether sugar is an "anti-nutrient", meaning that it requires a lot of water and it steals essential vitamins and minerals just to be digested. Sugar provides nothing of nutritional value, and requires other nutrients to be processed, in particular vitamin B1.[3] I personally consider sugar to be a major anti-nutrient. It's hard enough to get all of the nutrients that your body needs on a daily basis, it makes it almost impossible when the body has to spend its nutrient stores to digest sugar.

Sugar provides nothing of nutritional value

It's common knowledge to most holistic doctors and some MD's that soft drinks contribute to dehydration and poor health. This fact must have escaped most of the modern medical community. Have you ever spent time in a hospital? Most people that I know in the hospital are dehydrated, and have IV fluids going into their arms. All you have to do is ask for a soft drink and one will be delivered to you soon by a nurse or an assistant. Does this make sense? The place we go to when we are very sick will routinely bring you a man-made beverage that is notorious for causing general bad health and dehydration. Oh but don't worry, there is the diet soft drink variety, in case you are a diabetic. Are you kidding me? They are even worse! Aspartame and sucralose will be discussed at length in chapter 6. It is all maddening. This should be a teaching moment for the doctors and nurses. Here is this sick captive audience that should be taught the importance of proper hydration. This rarely if ever happens. They are served up the very thing that has potentially contributed to their general health problems, perhaps even the problem that they are in the hospital for requiring IV fluids.

I understand when patients feel bad they should be comforted when possible. At the very least, have the dehydration discussion with the patient. I have never heard a doctor discuss the health problems, or dehydration caused by soft drinks in a hospital or an office setting. A lot of the very same nurses that will bring you these soft drinks are drinking Coke, Mountain Dew, Red Bull, Monster, Amp, or some other soda or energy drink to keep them awake or energized. From my vast observational experiences in hospitals with my mother, many (not all) nurses are also dehydrated, significantly overweight, and under nourished.

While visiting a patient in a local hospital, I saw a picture and name of that hospital on the front panel of the soft drink and junk food vending machines in the E.R. waiting room. This hospital did not hide their affiliation with these products that are contributing so much to our poor health. I feel sure that the hospital is sharing in the profits from the sale of these drinks as well. I know it is unrealistic to expect vending machines filled with broccoli, free range eggs, purified water, and non GMO fruits and veggies in them.

The soft drink issue is just one thing that re-affirms my position that hospitals are not places of wellness and health. Hospitals are full of wonderful caring hard working nurses, doctors, kitchen staff, maintenance, and housekeeping workers, etc. Having spent countless days and nights in the hospital with my mother, my family and I know how caring most of these people are. My larger point here is that hospitals are for emergencies and interventions, not health and wellness.

I asked one of the hospital dining room supervisors about some of my issues with soft drinks, hot dogs, French fries, foods with all kinds of additives like monosodium glutamate (MSG), and nutra-sweet (now called Amino-Sweet), various preservatives, potato chips, and other unhealthy things available at a so called health institution. Her response was very interesting to me. She said that people will not select the healthier options; they tried putting healthy selections in their menu, but most of it was wasted and thrown away at the end of the day. So basically the hospitals are a reflection, a microcosm if you will, of our society at large. The same can be said for our public schools as I have a patient that is in charge of the menu at a local school. She communicated the same problem to me. Most school aged children will not choose the healthier options from the serving lines and they end up throwing most of it out.

This most unhealthy way of eating that I call the Standard American Diet (SAD) is so pervasive that it has to be made available to the public at hospitals and to our children in our public schools. It is a SAD but true reality indeed (pun intended).

Sugary treats and soft drinks have become so common in our daily lives, that we are literally addicted to them. Sugar is a very addictive substance. Alcohol is a pure carbohydrate. So people addicted to sugar and people who are alcoholics suffer from very similar addictions. Where are the endocrinologists? Where are the nutritionists in our modern health care system on this?

In the late 90's I was invited by a local hospital to participate in a health fair they were conducting. They placed me next to a hospital "nutritionist". She was drinking a diet drink and was considerably overweight. She was handing out pamphlets touting the benefits of Olestra, a sucrose polyester type of man-made oil that was developed by Proctor and Gamble in 1968 and approved for snack foods in the mid 90's. What happened to Olestra and "Wow" chips, and fat free Pringles? They have seemingly disappeared! I got into a rather loud argument with the hospital "nutritionist" over the crap advice she was giving. Since I was not really there with the hospital group, they moved me under the stairs, go figure. When are we going to wake up to the reality that nutrition is not on the top burner in our modern health care system?

During the writing of this book, I was asked to co-produce and participate in a natural health seminar to employees at a local nursing home. My friend and I worked several hours on the information that we presented. Most of the attendees were overweight and mostly uninterested in the subject material. Several of them were clinging to their Diet Mountain Dews, obviously the beverage of choice among the nurses and assistants as they contain more caffeine than most other soft drinks. Many of the fatigued and overweight attendees sat in the back and talked a lot during the presentation and were poking fun at our material. There were a lot of empty seats in the front of the room and several of the attendees were asleep in their chairs during our presentation. We covered many subjects like excess consumption of sugars and sugary treats and refined foods, especially wheat products. We gave solutions for some common dietary problems and misconceptions. All throughout the program we asked if anyone had questions about our topics; there were only three or four questions over a two hour presentation. In the background a disoriented patient continuously called out "Nurse, nurse, help me". This went on the entire two hours we were there and the attendants were totally oblivious to it.

I felt like I was in a time warp or something. I didn't have a good feeling about what I was witnessing. All I could think of is how precious our health is. The employees of this facility seemed so unaware as to why the people they work with are so sick. There should have been dozens of questions and people clamoring for quality information, but that was not the case. All these people wanted to do was get credit for attending the in-house presentation and then go home.

When I have patients seeking true wellness, the first thing I require them to do is give up soft drinks and replace them with pure water. If I did nothing else for them, I have just increased their lifespan and improved the quality of their life. Diabetics in particular have no business drinking soft drinks of any kind, especially the diet drinks. If you are a diabetic, hello, you have a sugar problem. Most people do not know that diet drinks stimulate your appetite, not exactly what a diabetic needs. Everyone of the diabetics in my office has been told by their doctors that they should choose diet drinks over the regular ones. I tell them NO SOFT DRINKS OF ANY KIND!!!!! I just can't be more clear on this. If a patient just cannot do without them, then they are addicted to them, either physically or emotionally and in almost every case they are dehydrated.

The sweetener most often used in the non-diet soft drinks is high fructose corn syrup (HFCS). This sweetener is notorious for increasing triglyceride levels.[3] It contributes to overall inflammation and therefore is a major player in the development of cardiovascular disease. Understand we are not talking about a fat here, we are talking about a sugar. HFCS is one of the by-products of the massive use of corn in this country and it is cheaper than cane sugar. A great book on the history of corn in America is The Omnivores Dilemma, by Michael Pollan.[4] Mr. Pollans' book comes in two varieties, one that's hard hitting and has some strong language in it, and another one that is good for a younger audience.

White table sugar (sucrose) is composed of two different sugar molecules glucose and fructose. Glucose is a primary fuel for our bodies. Fructose is the sugar that is very easily converted into triglycerides. High fructose corn syrup contains 55% fructose, table sugar contains 50% fructose, not that much difference. While high fructose corn syrup is bad, table sugar is not much better. Excess consumption of simple refined sugars in any form increases inflammation and is converted into body fat or triglycerides. Chronic inflammation is a major cause of poor health, particularly heart disease. If you really want to reduce your risk of heart disease and reduce your triglycerides, eliminate sugars! Find out where the hidden sugars are in your diet and start to eliminate them totally.

Honey and maple syrup are not sugar substitutes, they are sugar. It's just that they are in different forms. Because they are simple sugars they are rapidly assimilated into the bloodstream, they are not allowed on the program for that reason. These simple sugars cause a rapid insulin response. Remember, the excess sugars in the bloodstream are primarily converted into triglycerides. Anything that causes insulin to respond in an excessive manner is not good for you. The lower you can keep your insulin production over your lifetime, the healthier you will be. Honey does have some benefits in the natural health world. For example, it works well to reduce the pain of fever blisters around the mouth, (just dab it on the fever blister several times a day). Local bee pollen can have some benefit to people suffering with seasonal allergies (start taking it about two weeks before the allergy season arrives). Bee pollen must not be taken by people who have allergies to bee stings.

The lower you can keep your insulin production over your life time, the healthier you will be.

A common source of hidden refined sugars is breakfast cereals. It's typical in America to start our children's morning off with a highly refined wheat cereal loaded with chemicals and food colorings. Most of these cereals are coated in sugar from the manufacturer. Often the children are allowed to put more sugar on the cereal before it is covered with some highly processed milk. Is it any wonder they have trouble paying attention in school? They are either bouncing off the wall from the refined sugars, and/or suffering from the exhaustion caused by two of the most common food allergies in America (wheat and processed dairy). They could be KooKo from Coco Puffs, loopy from Fruit Loops, or too pooped to pop after eating Pop Tarts. They can't pay attention and are often diagnosed with ADD or ADHD, when it's really just their diets. Many of these children are put on the ADD/ADHD drugs like Ritalin or Adderall, to help them pay attention in school. Ritalin and cocaine have similar chemical structures, and addictive properties.[5]

By teaching families how to eat correctly, a lot of parents are able to get their children off of Ritalin and other ADD drugs, by simply changing their diets. Again a good book to suggest to you here is *Gut and Psychology Sydrome* by Dr. Natasha Campbell-McBride MD. Her program is called the GAPS diet.[6] I highly recommend it if you, or one of your children, has an attention problem. The program requires some effort, but is very effective in helping with learning disabilities and autism. Another fabulous book on ADD and ADHD is- *Is This Your Child,* by Doris Rapp

MD.(7) It is a big book but well worth the read if you have a child that is very combative, will not mind, or has been labeled with ADD or ADHD. It's highly possible that these children do not have "conditions" or a "disease", they have unidentified food sensitivities or food allergies.

There are plenty of hidden sources of sugars or high fructose corn syrup. A good example is ketchup, some children, and a lot of adults, smother their foods in ketchup. I have watched this in local eateries and when I am traveling. It's common to see children smothering their breakfast potatoes with ketchup on the same plate with refined wheat pancakes covered with imitation maple syrup made from high fructose corn syrup. They swallow this down with some chocolate milk, soda or juice. Most parents are unaware of what this does to their children. If parents are unaware of the detrimental effects of eating this way for their children, then they have no clue of what they are doing to their own health. Families that eat this way together, get sick together. I call this familial disease. We learn most of our eating habits from our parents.

One thing that really upsets me is watching an infant drink from a bottle that has a soft drink in it.

One thing that really upsets me is watching an infant drink from a bottle that has a soft drink in it. This is how we have become a sugar addicted nation. Where has our common sense gone? It is beyond me how millions of people can't see this. If you watch television on Saturday mornings with your children, you will see ad after ad for these sugary cereals and treats. You have to know the food industry is not going to step up to the plate and do what's right. So after ten, twenty, or thirty years of this behavior, these infants that are now adults develop multiple health problems. They show up in an office like mine seeking magic solutions. Where has the responsibility of the food industry been? Where have the doctors and dietitians been all these years? You cannot count on doctors, corporations, advertisers, news agencies, or our government to give you health. Staying healthy (here it comes) is your responsibility.

Most of the patients I see that are seeking health advice have back pain, are overweight, on high blood pressure medicines, many of them take something to help them sleep. They drink some form of caffeine in the mornings to get them going. A good many of them are taking statin drugs for their cholesterol. Some are taking warfarin (a rat poison) to keep their blood viscosity at a certain point. Many of them suffer with arthritis, gout, fibromyalgia, hypertension, skin problems, bad breath, irritable bowels, constipation or diarrhea or both, ringing in their ears, and a hundred more things I could mention. I always ask them how much water they drink, and how much sugar they consume. It's amazing to me how many people do not drink any water and have no idea how much sugar they eat. Hidden sugars/carbohydrates along with the obvious ones really mount up over a day's time.

Just before sitting down to write this chapter, I went to see a friend of mine. He had just pulled some lasagna out of the oven. He asked me if I wanted to eat some supper. I explained that I had already had supper. I watched him drink two Pepsi colas (80 plus grams of carbohydrates), 3 slices of highly processed white bread covered in margarine (45 grams of carbohydrates, and some hydrogenated fat), not to mention the carbs he got from the wheat noodles in the lasagna. I estimated about 150 grams of carbohydrate in one meal. I told him about it and he just shrugged his shoulders and said, "I eat like this all the time". This is how we have become addicted to sugars. We are clueless.

Our primary mainstream sources for health information are doctors, nutritionists, dietitians, nurses, schools, the media, health institutions, and the food industry. Also in the mix is the biased, for profit, drug commercials plastered all over our TV screens (and soon after, the law suits over those drugs). All combined, one has to conclude that these institutions have failed us. I also know some alternative practitioners that give poor dietary and nutritional advice.

Cancer has a particular affinity to sugar.(10) There is even some good evidence that a diet high in refined carbohydrates (especially high fructose corn syrup) can actually contribute to developing cancer over time.(9) Some of my patients who have cancer tell me that their oncologists have told them that eating sugar is not a problem. This always makes me wonder just how much of their own research practicing physicians actually read. A good book on this subject is *The Hidden Story Of Cancer,* by Brian Scott Peskin, BSEE.(10) This book chronicles the life and works of Otto Warburg, who did an incredible body of research in the early 1900's; his results have been largely ignored by the medical profession. It is a good book to read if you are interested in how to help yourself from ever developing cancer. Dr. Warburg spoke extensively on increased fermentation processes in the body fueled by sugar. Mr. Peskin writes:

> Dr. Warburg always considered the ratio of increased fermentation, to decreased respiration as the prime characteristic of cancer cells. (11)

So if cancer prevention is something that is of interest to you, first give up sugar, wheat, and junk foods. Then examine your chemical exposure in your home and at work. Start reading some of the books I have suggested to you. Be proactive.

If you have been diagnosed with cancer it is fairly common to have a Positron Emission Tomography (PET) scan to determine where the cancer is in your body. These PET scans are done using a radiographic isotope and sugar.(12) The sugar helps the isotope gain entrance into the cancer cells as cancer has a real affinity for sugar, it thrives on it. So for the medical profession to ignore the sugar connection to cancer is insane. Sugar feeds cancer and promotes the fermentation Dr. Warburg warned about.

Nutrition is never the topic of conversation in the traditional oncology office as far as I can see. I know this because I always ask my patients with cancer about it. They say their doctors tell them diet doesn't make any difference. Recently, one of my patients and his wife were at the oncologist's office for his appointment. The staff offered them a Coke and a Krispy Kreme donut while they were waiting. Wisely, they declined the offer because I had educated them on the cancer/sugar connection. Traditional oncologists place no importance on the relationship of sugar or diet in general as it relates to cancer. This is slowly changing. I see the advertisements for the Cancer Treatment Centers of America on television; they advertise that a nutritional counselor is on your "team". I don't know what kind of nutritional advice they give or how much weight nutrition is given in the overall treatment. At the least it's a move in the right direction, but I am skeptically optimistic.

You need to limit your exposure to sugar. It would be optimal if it could be totally eliminated, but this is very hard to do. There is a lot of science out there about sugar, simple vs. complex, refined vs. raw, diagrams of the molecular structure, and so on. I could spend a lot of time and paper here going into great detail about sugar and what it does in the body. This is not meant to be a physiology book, it is meant to be a starting point for you. Trust me here and try to limit your total carbohydrate intake to between 50 and 100 grams a day (75 grams is the sweet spot.) If you are a diabetic, it is very important to keep close tabs on the changes in your blood sugar levels. The results will be obvious to you very quickly if you take my advice. Don't be surprised if giving up sugar takes several weeks to do. Using lemon in your water in the mornings can help to reduce your sugar cravings. If you would like to read a classic book about sugar, *The Sugar Blues,* by William Dufty[13] is a great one to pick up, and covers the history of sugar very comprehensively. This was truly one of the most informative and entertaining books I ever read.

My second cousin is disabled and needs assistance to get her groceries and toiletries every month or so. She likes to go to one of the local big box stores so she can get everything she needs. We were at the store at the first of the month when the disability and government checks went out and she was tooling around in one of those motorized carts getting her things. We went to check out and in front of us was a guy also on one of the motorized carts checking out. The motorized carts have small baskets and don't hold much merchandise. He had his son with him who also had another regular cart full of things that his father was purchasing. As they were checking out, I couldn't help but notice the items purchased by this man with his monthly check.

The outer part of the cages on both carts, were lined with six packs of diet drink cartons that had been draped over the edges. Inside the cart were several packets of prescription drugs from the pharmacy. Also in the cart were donuts, candy bars, pop tarts, jellies, all types of breads, hot dogs, bologna, TV dinners, many boxes of cereals, cakes, pies, 1% low fat milk, crackers, and peanut butter. Well you get the point. I didn't see any quality food in either of those two carts, no lean cuts of meats, absolutely no fresh fruits or vegetables. It was all empty carbs, diet drinks, and chemically laden processed foods. What really got to me was that this man was probably 400 lbs. or more, he was using an oxygen line, had skin conditions, his ankles were very swollen, and he was obviously in very poor health. The final striking observation for me was the pack of cigarettes in his front pocket and he looked to be in his early fifties, a young man by my standard. I don't know the entire story behind this guy, and I certainly am not passing judgment on him. Maybe he made these purchases because he lives alone and these packaged foods are easy to prepare.

This is not the first time I have seen someone like him in that store. Sadly, there are a lot of people in poor health riding around in those carts. Most of them have similar things in their buggies. I know you have seen this too. I would like to be able to talk to all of them in the presence of their doctors and families. Other than obvious traumas, I would like to know what it was that created or allowed their situations to develop. It's hard for me to understand why some people can't see that they caused and continue to perpetuate their health conditions. Perhaps they have just given up. I would like to let them know that they may be able to improve their situations with the right information mixed with some hope and inspiration. Maybe you or one of your family members is in this situation.

The common thread in this scenario is the types of foods in the buggies. It was mainly dead, high wheat and grain content, chemically laden, high sugar, highly processed, cheap foods. There are usually always several bags of medicines in there from the pharmacy. They are all overweight, a lot of them on oxygen, and some of them are obviously still smoking. Even folks that have declined to this point can, over time, make significant changes to their health given the right advice. The reality is that most of them will never know. This is what frustrates me the most as I know that I could probably help them, but much like my own family, I cannot place my values on people that are not ready for it or didn't ask for it. I don't really know why I wanted to mention this other than it is important to look around at how unhealthy we Americans really are. I am very sad for those people. Most of them are truly suffering from the "sugar blues".

Complex sugars are found mainly in non-starchy vegetables and grains. These foods contain generally contain more fiber along with multiple sugars linked together that must be broken down before they can be absorbed. This is why quality non-starchy vegetables are at the foundation of the REGENESIS dietary program.

The main difference in complex and simple or refined sugars is how fast they are released into the body. Simple sugars are released quickly and absorbed very fast. Complex sugars are released slower because the body has to work to break them down. The effects are obvious as simple sugars cause a rapid response of insulin by the body and the complex sugars cause a much slower gradual response. The slower response is more desirable.

Vegetables can provide us with a good example of the differences in carbohydrates. In some vegetables like potatoes, carbohydrates are more easily released than the carbohydrates in a vegetable like celery. For people with blood sugar issues, they know that a baked potato will raise their blood sugar levels very quickly; almost as fast as a candy bar or orange juice. Celery on the other hand has a more complex sugar along with fiber and causes little to no insulin response from the body. The message here is that the complex carbohydrates are better for you if you are overweight, tired, or a diabetic.

The Glycemic Index

The Glycemic Index estimates how much each gram of available carbohydrate (total carbohydrate minus fiber) in a food raises a persons' blood glucose level following consumption of the food relative to the consumption of pure glucose. (14)

The glycemic index helps in sorting out better food choices. It serves you better to eat foods that are lower on the glycemic index as opposed to the ones high on the list. For example, corn flakes are on the list at 89, lentils are on the list at 29. Based on glycemic index values, lentils are a much better choice than corn flakes. This is how you would use the glycemic index to make better food choices in regards to your total carbohydrate intake.

You can pull up the glycemic index online, or if you want to know the total carbohydrates, fats, or protein content of any food, just Google it if you have a computer. It's good to educate yourself on how many grams of carbohydrates you are consuming per day.

Refined sugar and fruit sugar are simple sugars but there are stark differences. Refined sugars are just that, they have been refined; they are not in their natural state. The sugars in whole fruits are still intact in the fruit and must be digested in order for your body to have access to them. It's better to eat a piece of fruit than it is to eat the equivalent amount of refined sugars; at least the fruit has some beneficial nutrients in it. If you have sugar issues or are trying to lose weight, it's best to avoid simple sugars period (pardon the redundancy). If you are a diabetic, it makes no sense to eat anything containing simple sugars. It always amazes me at how much fruit and carbohydrates are allowed in a diabetic diet that has been provided by dietitians, nutritionists, and the American Diabetic Association.

If you are a diabetic, it makes no sense to eat anything containing simple sugars.

> One of my diabetic patients told me that when she was first diagnosed, she attended a program on diet given by a dietitian/nutritionist. The cost of the class was $2400.00, her insurance paid for the class. She was instructed to eat at least 45 grams of carbohydrates with each meal. I am perplexed by this logic. She said that they did not really differentiate what kinds of carbohydrates were allowed. She had been eating this way for some time and it was no surprise to me that her sugar issues had not improved in the least. After ten weeks on the REGENESIS plan, her A1C (a long term blood sugar measurement) dropped under the diabetic range. Her fasting blood sugars were down 25 plus points. In ten months, she lost over one hundred pounds. She is feeling a lot better overall but there is even more improvement in her future if she remains on the REGENESIS program.

Strawberries, blueberries, blackberries, pomegranites, and raspberries are allowed on the program (1 cup a day). These berries are rich in powerful phytonutrients called anthocyanins. These phytonutrients are responsible for the deep blue, purple and red colors of the colorful fruits and vegetables. They help reduce the inflammation associated with coronary heart disease (CHD), and they are beneficial for people with retina problems, ulcers, and allergies. Berries are rich in antioxidants. Strawberries tend to take up pesticides very easily, making the organically grown berries much more preferable. When deciding which fruits and veggies to eat, always chose a wide variety of colors to take advantage of the bountiful antioxidant value found in these colorful foods.

Wheat products, refined and whole wheat, are very high on the glycemic index and must absolutely be avoided by diabetics and people trying to lose weight, or by anyone that wants to be healthy. One slice of white bread can contain up to the equivalent of 4 teaspoons of white sugar! White flour is a refined food that is not in the natural state. Your body has much easier access to the sugars after a food has been refined. Spaghetti noodles, breads of all kinds, pizza crusts, and cereals must be avoided if you want to recapture your health. The old food pyramid suggested up to 11 servings of grains a day. This is crazy. I would suggest to you NO servings of grains per day (I told you I would give you a contrarian opinion). People look at me funny when I tell them to give up breads. It is so engrained into our eating habits (you had to see that one coming). The ones that do give up their breads and grains notice very quickly how much better they feel and how much more energy they have. Many report significant decreases in stiffness, joint pain, fatigue, and a general improvement in mental function and attitude.

Complex sugars found in non-starchy vegetables are the primary and preferred source of carbohydrates on the REGENESIS program. These vegetables have multiple carbon chains that must be broken down into glucose, which is the form of sugar used by your body. The larger the carbon chain, the harder your body has to work to break them down, therefore the slower the release of glucose. When this happens your body has longer to deal with the sugar released, and the response of insulin is slower and consequently not as large as when simple sugars are consumed (I know I keep going over and over this, but it's so important). Along with the carbohydrate in the vegetables, there are minerals, fiber, enzymes, vitamins, amino acids, and other beneficial nutrients that are used by the body. Contrast this to refined sugars that do not have any of the beneficial nutrients of a whole food. The complex carbohydrates are preferable, and simple refined carbohydrates must be avoided.

Vegetables that have the least amount of sugars and the highest amounts of beneficial nutrients are the best choices. Lettuces, cruciferous vegetables like broccoli and cauliflower, onions, peppers (all colors), and all types of squash are good choices. Vegetables that contain higher content of sugars are the starchy carbohydrates, mainly beans and potatoes. On the REGENESIS program, non-starchy vegetables are preferred over the starchy vegetables. Did I just say that again? This keeps the insulin response of the body at a minimum, which is one of the main goals of the program. For that reason, stay away from table sugars, fruits, fruit juices, high fructose corn syrup, white potatoes, wheat products, and breads of all kinds. As discussed in the previous chapter on wheat, there are many reasons to avoid wheat and this is just another one.

One of my primary goals here (especially if you are diabetic), is to help you understand the differences between different types of sugars and why you should avoid excess consumption of sugars in general. The less insulin your body produces in your lifetime, the healthier you will be and the longer you will live. You have a general guideline for which kinds of foods to eat and the kinds to avoid (see the Eating Guidelines, chapter 12). It will be important for you to know how to read food labels, we will go over this topic in chapter 11 (the leftovers chapter).

Dr. Diana Schwarzbein was one of the first doctors I ever heard speak on hidden sugars. She talked about how the traditional diabetic diets recommended by doctors and dietitians are incorrect. She wrote a great book called *The Schwarzbein Principle* (15), it was one of the first books I ever read on the subject of correcting or substantially improving diabetic issues with diet.

She pointed out that prolonged high insulin levels led to "accelerated metabolic aging" which increases body fat and degenerative conditions seen in diabetics (kidney, heart, vascular and others). She spoke of the factors that directly or indirectly raise insulin levels such as medications (prescription and over the counter), lack of exercise, alcohol consumption, stress, artificial sweetener use and others. She suggested that the increase in these factors paralleled the increased incidences of diabetes from around 1980 to 1999. (16)

Her comments are spot on. Her book was published in 1999 but nothing has really changed as I have not seen a significant shift in suggestions or recommendations regarding diet from the medical profession. It seems the high grain content, low to no saturated fat, low cholesterol "prudent diet" is all they really know how to recommend. Many doctors, including endocrinologists, consume and recommend artificial sweeteners to diabetics. This is crazy in light of all the credible information there is out there about the harmful effects of these food additives.

I highly recommend that you eat some raw foods every day. Some vegetables are delicious raw once you get use to eating them. Eat a fresh salad made with some raw veggies daily if possible as they are loaded with antioxidants, enzymes, and minerals. Use lemon or lime juice on salads instead of oil based dressings (the taste will surprise you). Raw sweet potatoes are delicious and make a great snack.

Squash is one of the foods being genetically modified more and more, so I highly suggest that if you eat squash, that it is non GMO and organic. Non starchy vegetables are great for making soups. This is a great way to use left-over veggies and not waste portions that may be too small to constitute a meal.

I highly recommend that you eat some raw foods every day.

Just for reference, 4 grams of sugar equals 1 teaspoon. Some breads contain 16 grams of sugar (carbohydrates) per slice, that's 4 teaspoons of sugar for one slice of bread! Anything that contains over 8 grams of sugar will spike your insulin levels. Fruit filled sweetened yogurt has around 30 grams of carbohydrate, that is almost 8 teaspoons of sugar.

Giving up simple sugars, watching total carbohydrate consumption, eliminating grains from the diet, and proper hydration through adequate water consumption will cause a significant shift in your overall health. Add complex carbohydrates with the non-starchy veggies, and eat raw foods daily. These things alone are generally enough to start you on the way to losing weight if you have a weight problem. These changes usually start to put some energy into your energy bank as well.

There are numerous other sweeteners not explained in this section. None of them are allowed on the plan. They include brown rice syrup, date sugars, turbinado sugar, agave, and barley malt syrup. When it comes to sweeteners, there simply is no "savior "out there. If you need to sweeten things, you must find some quality pure stevia drops (alcohol free is preferred) and learn how to use them (I use about 4 drops to a glass of lemonade). Once you learn to eat quality foods, you will feel a lot better, and your sweet tooth will be easily satisfied by mother natures' pure foods. If you just can't move past this, you may be allergic to sugar, or you are eating out of an emotional need for pleasure. As stated before, if you are eating emotionally, it requires that you do some soul searching and identify why. Depak Chopara has written a wonderful book called *What Are You Hungry For,* it can help you identify your emotional eating problem. Make the necessary changes in your life so you can move forward in your quest for health.

5

Oils, Fats, and Cholesterol

"American consumers have no problem with carcinogens, but they will not purchase any product, including floor wax, that has fat in it"
Dave Barry

THERE HAS BEEN a lot of discussion about oils, fats, and cholesterol, a lot of it true, a lot of it not so true. How does one know what is the truth and what is fiction? It is my hope that after you read this chapter you will be clear on the importance of quality oils, fats, and yes, <u>quality cholesterol consumption</u>. Again, it is your responsibility to dig deeper if you need to know more. I have recommended some good sources in this chapter for you.

For our discussion here, oils are mostly man-made, fats (also called fatty acids) are naturally occurring substances found in plants and animals. Cholesterol is an oily waxy like substance also found in plants and animals and is crucial for human health. If you're not sure where you stand on this topic, let me ask you a few questions:

* Are you following your doctor's advice?
* Are you eating your recommended amounts of whole grains?
* Are you using cholesterol-free cooking oils and margarine?

* Are you following the food pyramid recommendations by avoiding saturated fats?

If so, your cholesterol should be perfect, right? You should be at your ideal body weight, correct? You should not have high blood pressure. If you are doing the things mentioned above, then how did you get to this point? Obviously, if things were perfect, you wouldn't be reading a book about recovering your health.

One hundred years ago, Americans were not plagued by heart disease, cancer, diabetes, and osteoporosis. Alzheimer's disease was not a consideration fifty years ago.[1] Dr. Paul Dudley White, the founder of modern day cardiology, who graduated from Harvard medical school was quoted as saying: "When I graduated from medical school in 1911, I had never heard of a coronary thrombosis" (heart attack). [2]

Years ago, Americans were not plagued by heart disease, cancer, diabetes, and osteoporosis.

Corn oil was invented in 1911 by a company called Mazola. Crisco was invented by Proctor and Gamble in the same year. I went to the Crisco website and found this statement:

> "Crisco is the first shortening product made entirely of vegetable oil, was the result of hydrogenation, a new process that produced shortening that would stay in solid form year-round, regardless of temperature". [3]

Hydrogenation in the early 1900's changed everything and Americans were consuming more foods cooked in man-made processed fats. Shortly after the invention of these hydrogenated fats, heart attacks began increasing to the point that in 1920, at Massachusetts General Hospital, the afore mentioned Dr. Paul Dudley White, initiated an entire new branch of medicine called Cardiology. I don't know of one sane person that would argue that hydrogenated man-made fats are a good thing for our health.

How did we get so fearful of essential cholesterol? Why is naturally occurring cholesterol perceived as bad? What are good oils? What should we be eating? What should we be cooking our foods in? All of the preceding questions are reasonable questions. How do we arrive at the truth? Perhaps we should look backwards to see how we got here.

One of the first pioneers who sounded the alarm about processed foods was a dentist from Cleveland, Ohio, named Dr. Weston A. Price. His foundation headed by Sally Fallon, is still around and challenges today's politically correct dietary recommendations from who she calls the "diet dictocrats". Dr. Price started to notice a lot more dental and other health problems in people that were consuming refined foods like sugars and white flour products. Dr. Price termed these foods "foods for commerce". [4]

Dr. Price and his wife traveled to several countries all over the world for over ten years. He studied many populations including tribal Africans, Pacific islanders, Eskimos, Melanesians and Polynesians, North and South American natives, Inuit, and Australian Aborigines and Malay tribes. He studied generations of remote tribal people and took numerous photographs of healthy and unhealthy individuals including their teeth and compared his dental exam findings. He observed natives that had been removed from tribal ancestral dietary traditions he called them "modernized natives". These "modernized natives" were consuming modern processed foods including sugars and refined grains. He documented the rapid and profound downward health spiral he witnessed in these people.

His comparative findings were very convincing that processed foods were indeed causing multiple health problems. Modernized natives that were consuming refined products had more problems with dental cavities, alignment of teeth, dental arch formation, disease resistance (TB in particular), general health, behavioral problems, and developmental issues.[5] Dr. Price wrote about his findings in one of the first books about the problems with these new processed foods, *Nutrition and Physical Degeneration*.[6] The book is a classic and is a little difficult to read but well worth the effort.

The Weston A. Price Foundation website is a great source for information. I highly suggest you spend some time there reading some of the articles. If you are looking for a very informative weekend, attend one of their seminars. Their website is- *www.westonaprice.org*

From an article written on Dec. 26, 2005, Sally Fallon the president of the Weston A. Price Foundation writes:

> "Weston A. Price, DDS, discovered that as populations adopt processed foods, with each generation the facial structure becomes more and more narrow. Healthy faces should be broad. We are all designed to have perfectly straight teeth and not get cavities. When you are eating real, nutrient-dense foods, you get the complete and perfect expression of the genetic potential. We were given a perfect blueprint. Whether or not the body temple is built according to the blueprint, to a great extent, on our wisdom in food choices.
>
> To be healthy, we need to prepare our own food, for ourselves and for our families. This doesn't mean you have to spend hours in the kitchen, but you do need to spend some time there, preparing food with wisdom and love. If no one in the family has time to prepare food, you need to sit down and rethink how you are spending your time, because this is the only way to get nourishing foods into your children. We can return to good eating practices one mouth at a time, one meal at a time, by preparing our own food and preparing it properly." [7]

There have been many others who have sounded alarms on the food industry, but few have heeded their warnings. With the advent of fast foods, and both parents working, it was a convenient and easy transition for folks to make as foods became faster and easier to prepare. During this explosion of packaged and fast foods, people, especially mothers, were bombarded with TV commercials and magazine advertisements.

The problem was that, along with this convenience came processing, food additives, preservatives, and packaging. No longer were families cooking at home like before. Quality time around the family dinner table began to erode, as the fast food lifestyle was becoming more of a part of our culture.

Fast food joints started popping up in the late 50's and early 60's. Some of them are still in existence today and at the same locations. America's obsession with waitresses on roller skates, rock-n-roll, cruising, fast foods, and fast hot rods, slicked back hair, pony tails, bobby socks, and penny loafers had begun. Now there are fast food places of all types on every corner. A great book I want to suggest to you here is *Fast Food Nation* [8], by Eric Schlosser. A great documentary to watch on this subject is *Super Size Me* [9], by Morgan Spurlock. This documentary about how fast foods are making us sick and obese can be rented from your favorite rental store or watched online.

Also springing up were the diseases of convenience: increasing heart disease, cancer, diabetes, obesity, fibromyalgia, arthritis, neurological diseases, and many others. The major shift here was the use of man-made hydrogenated fats replacing traditional naturally occurring fats along with ever increasing consumption of refined wheat, sugar products, and junk foods laced with chemicals.

The new so called "healthy" processed oils have become a real problem. These oils are not natural and the body does not know how to properly process and eliminate them. These fats are potentially rancid to begin with, mainly due to the manufacturing process. A rancid fat is one of, if not the worst things you can consume. They are a major source of free radicals, which will be covered in chapter eleven.

Before being sold to consumers, seed oils, soy, corn, and other vegetable oils are highly refined. Some of the last steps in this refining process involve hydrogenation (to make it a solid like margarine), bleaching, and deodorization. Deodorization is required in order to remove the smell of the rancid oils.[10] Oils become rancid because of the heat and light that they are exposed to during the manufacturing process and are rancid before they ever reach your home.

Below are some of the steps that seeds go through in order to be transformed into oils that are sold for human consumption:

EXPELLER PRESSING → SOLVENT EXTRACTION → DEGUMMING → CAUSTIC REFINING → BLEACHING → DEWAXING → FRACTIONATION → HYDROGENATION → POST BLEACHING → DEODORIZATION → PLASTICIZATION (11)

Highly refined oils are used heavily in the fast food industry as they are cheap and can be used for several days before they must be changed. Not only are corn, soy, canola, and cotton seed oils unhealthy, the seeds they come from are potentially genetically modified. Seed oils, like cottonseed oil and canola oil are processed in a similar fashion as vegetable oils. Margarine and shortening go through many of the same processes including bleaching, deodorization, hydrogenation, and plasticization. Canola oil, from the rapeseed plant, is one of the oils generally made from a highly genetically modified organism (GMO) seed. Unlike a lot of "experts", I do not recommend canola oil. By far the most commonly used oil used in America today is highly refined soy oil.(12)

Monsanto has discovered a way to modify genetic codes in order to make several of their crop seeds immune to Round Up, an herbicide that is manufactured by them. Farmers use these seeds, which allow them to saturate the crop with Round Up killing the weeds between the rows of crops. This eliminates manual methods of removing weeds and increases yield while reducing production costs. (13) The result is profits for Monsanto in seed and herbicide production, and increased profits for commercial farmers in reduced labor costs.

If you consume these GMO foods, you are eating from crops that have been hybridized, and/or genetically altered, then saturated with the herbicide Round Up. It matters what you put into your body (which is your temple) over your lifetime.

Cotton seeds are basically a waste product of the cotton industry.

One of the seed oils commonly used comes from cottonseed. Crisco is hydrogenated cottonseed oil. You will find cottonseed oil in a lot of cellophane packaged foods like peanuts, snack cakes, and many other food products. It is cheap, potentially rancid, and a source of free radicals. Cottonseed oil is not a natural food oil. When was the last time you had a plate of cotton for supper? Cotton seeds are basically a waste product of the cotton industry. Much like the corn industry, the cotton industry uses every last component of the crop to maximize profits (it's business, it's not health). The leftover seeds from cotton production are cheap and plentiful.

The Boll Weevil is the primary threat to cotton and the industry sprays the crops heavily with pesticides. The cotton industry is not held to the same standards for chemical use as the food industry. (14)

Cottonseed oil is processed in a similar fashion as other seed oils and the potential chemical contamination from pesticides and herbicides makes consumption of this oil highly problematic to me. I strongly advise my patients not to use cottonseed oil or any products that contain it (commonly found in packaged nuts). Obviously, the FDA has cleared cottonseed oil for human consumption. Do you trust the FDA and the food industry to protect your health?

The previously mentioned oils are some of the most common fats used in our modern food industry. There are others but hopefully you get the point. These processed oils are really the bad guys. They are often recommended for cooking because they are cholesterol free. Fats and oils that are found in nature can be easily processed by a healthy body. These include butter from raw milk fat, coconut oil, olive oil, beef tallow, and lard (yes, lard). These fats and oils have been used for centuries. When consumed in the proper amounts, and in the proper form, from organic plants, or from free ranging animals, they are actually healthy for you. Trillions of cells in your body are wrapped with a layer of cholesterol. Your brain is approximately 60% fats and cholesterol. Your hormones are mostly cholesterol by weight. You need fat and cholesterol. More appropriately stated, you need "quality" fat and cholesterol.

Think about it, would you want a brain nourished and supported by natural fats like butter, lard or coconut oil, or one composed and supported by hydrogenated vegetable oil from potato chips, donuts, or French fries? How many folks do you know that have hormone problems like low thyroid, PMS, erectile dysfunction, irregular menstrual cycles, endometriosis, cyclical related migraine headaches? Your body needs fats, oils, and cholesterol but they must be natural, unadulterated, quality fats. Some of the sickest people I have cared for over the years are the ones that are fearful of eating quality fats because of mis-information they have heard somewhere. They have stuck to reduced fat or fat free diets for years. Quality fats are essential to good health.

Some of the sickest people I have cared for over the years are the ones that are fearful of eating quality fats…

Some vegetarians are fat phobic and are lacking quality fats that are essential for maintaining a healthy body. It makes no difference to me if someone wants to practice a vegetarian lifestyle, but it's essential that they, as well as everyone else, supplement their diets to make up for what may be lacking nutritionally. I have helped some very sick vegetarians recapture their health by adding quality fats to their diets. Flax and hemp oils are in alignment with the vegetarian philosophy on animal fats. Good quality flax and hemp oils are easy to find.

Your body requires 90 or more nutrients every day, that's <u>every day</u> in order to be healthy. (15) It is virtually impossible now to get the required nutrients from our food supply. So if your health care provider says you can get all the nutrients you need from your food, he or she has been on vacation to Mars. Our own government (Senate document 264), recognized the general massive depletion of the minerals in our soils as far back as 1936! (16)

Corn, rice, and wheat make up approximately 80% of our food supply in America, 95% of what we eat today comes from only 30 crops. This was not the case before modern agricultural practices. Today commercial farming is done using seeds that have been adapted to create more yield (and understandably more profit). These farming practices discourage thousands of years of natural plant diversity. Often times, plants that are easier to grow, have better cosmetic qualities but contain much less in nutrient content. Over farming of soils year after year affect the nutritional value of commercially grown plants. It has been demonstrated that nutrient content of plants is superior when healthy topsoil is used to grow organic vegetables. The problem is that topsoil is being used up faster than it can be replenished.(17) Topsoil mineral depletion caused by our modern farming practices, is a major contributor to the poor health of our nation.

> I have a patient that is a hairdresser. She had been suffering with migraine headaches for years. Her doctors had followed all of the standard protocols for headaches. She was taking Maxaalt or other medications several times a week just so she could function. She was not enjoying a quality of life that she was working hard for. I treated her chiropractically and she improved a lot but she was still having some headaches. We started working on her diet and we have almost eradicated her headaches completely. I told her she needed to "change her oil", meaning she needed to start consuming quality fats, along with some other nutritional changes including proper vitamin and mineral supplementation. She has discontinued the use of traditional vegetable or seed based oils, in favor of the natural fats that I recommend to all of my patients. She has a lot more energy now, rarely has a headache and does not rely on medications to keep her going.

A new fear........CHOLESTEROPHOBIA

There is a new fear in America, created by the edible oils industry, politicians, and our medical institutions; I call it CHOLESTEROPHOBIA, the fear of your cholesterol numbers. This fear has become a national obsession. Cholesterol is a very controversial subject. The American mainstream healthcare institutions have bought into what is called the "lipid-hypothesis". Put plainly, the lipid-hypothesis is: If you eat saturated fats and cholesterol rich foods, it will clog your arteries and over time this creates coronary artery disease and atherosclerosis which, in turn, causes heart attacks and strokes.[18] There is virtually no <u>credible</u> research that backs up this over 60 year old theory initially put forth by Ancel Keys. [19]

A recent study published in Annals of Internal Medicine in March of 2014, refutes the idea that saturated fats cause coronary heart disease. The conclusion reads- "Current evidence does not clearly support cardiovascular guidelines that encourage high consumption of polyunsaturated fatty acids and low consumption of total saturated fats." [20]

When you dig down into the weeds, it is the un-natural processed fats, junk foods, stress/lifestyle, smoking, and consumption of refined wheat products and sugar that contribute most to heart disease and stroke. This one chapter alone will probably cause most conventionally trained doctors not to suggest this book, or maybe even demonize this book.

Remember, it is most likely your life choices, our modern food production and our overpriced chemical medicine based healthcare system that has you in poor health and reading these words to begin with. They have had their chance to help you for years, maybe even decades. How is that working? I am going to make some reading suggestions to you on this topic. The big cholesterol lie is so large I would have to write an entire book on the subject to explain it. Several quality books on cholesterol have already been written.

If we look at the big picture here, billions of dollars are spent on evaluating, and treating "high" cholesterol. There has been a very profitable new industry created around cholesterophobia. Tens of thousands of procedures, like stints, and bypass surgery, are done in the US every year. Almost everyone you talk to is taking a statin drug to lower their cholesterol numbers. Seventy five percent of people that have fatal heart attacks have normal cholesterol.[21] Heart disease is still the number one killer of Americans. Is this working? I don't think so. What could be the problem in our approach here? One place to look is the research and the way the research has been presented (manipulated), to get the public fearful of this new disease, cholesterophobia.

Have you seen the scary commercials? How about the one with the gurney following the guy around talking about the lurking heart attack he may have if he doesn't take the drug that is being advertised. This direct to consumer advertising makes us run to our doctors, demand the drug, get the prescription, and run to the nearest drug store (it seems there's one on every corner). The drug stores make you go past the beach balls, the candy, the cigarettes, junk foods, and the get well and sympathy cards before you can even get to the pharmacy counter.

All of the rhetoric, commercials, and ubiquitous standardized testing causes a lot of anxiety over cholesterol. I have patients that get very anxious and upset if their cholesterol numbers are over 200. Cholesterol numbers can fluctuate a great deal from day to day mostly in response to stress and or inflammation, not from consumption of quality natural fats.

When you take your pet to the vet, does he check its cholesterol? Why not? It is because veterinarians know this is not a good marker for determining the health of your pet. Cholesterol is the messenger, it is not the problem. Pets get perfect nutrition if their owners purchase quality pet foods. The animal food scientists and veterinarians have significantly extended the lives of our pets through proper nutritional formulas found in most pet foods. Quality pet foods have virtually eliminated our pet's inflammation response from food sources. Inflammation is one of the major factors in elevating cholesterol levels. Has your vet ever told you not to feed your dog table scraps? We eat foods that will cause our pets to be unhealthy, or could kill them. Think about that one.

Dr. Joel Wallach has authored one of the most comprehensive books ever written on animal nutrition. It is at the Smithsonian institute where we keep our national treasures. He makes the point that over 900 diseases in animals have been cured using nutrition [22]. Livestock animals do not have health insurance or health care like people do. If they did, a pound of beef from a cow with health insurance would cost $250.00. Veterinarians had to figure out long ago how to cure diseases in animals using pre and post conception nutrition. I make the point again that humans have not been so fortunate.

One of the most quoted studies ever done on cholesterol is the Framingham study, named after the town of Framingham, Mass. The problem with the study is that the data was manipulated to give the results desired, not necessarily the truth.

Years after the Framingham study, the director of the study, Dr. William Castelli, said- *"In Framingham, Massachusetts, the more saturated fat one ate, the more cholesterol one ate, the more calories one ate, the lower people's serum cholesterol …we found that the people who ate the most cholesterol, ate the most saturated fat, ate the most calories weighed the least and were the most physically active."* [23]

George Mann, ScD, MD, Former Co-Director, Framingham Study said- *"The diet-heart hypothesis has been repeatedly shown to be wrong, and yet, for complicated reasons of pride, profit, and prejudice, the hypothesis to be exploited by scientists, fund-raising enterprises, food companies and even governmental agencies. The public is being deceived by the greatest health scam of the century."* [24]

Numerous other studies on cholesterol have been done and the results were not accurately represented to the public or obviously to health care providers. I say "obviously" here because after sixty years of countless studies that do not support current dietary recommendations, we are still being told the same old lie regarding fats and oils. A great new book about the meta analysis of old studies that shows how we have been deceived regarding essential fats is *The Big Fat Lie* by Nina Teicholz.[25] She does a great job of explaining the politics, the motives behind the "Prudent diet", and the great deception regarding the role of saturated fats and cholesterol on our health.

Consuming proper amounts of <u>quality</u> saturated fats from animal or tropical plant sources, does not cause heart disease. It is the replacement of quality saturated fats with grains, junk carbohydrates and man-made fats and chemicals that contributes the most to the dietary causes of cardiovascular diseases. [26, 27]

There was a lot of politicking going on here. It has taken decades of false assertions by institutions that stand to make a lot of money to create cholesterophobia. Very profitable drugs were being developed and the bogus guidelines for their use were being contrived by these manipulated studies.[28] That is a pretty bold statement. I suggest you read about it for yourself, don't just believe me. A great place to start would be reading the online article, "The Oiling Of America" by Mary Enig and Sally Fallon. One of my favorite books on this vast topic is, *The Great Cholesterol Con*, by Anthony Colpo. One thing that really stuck with me while reading the book by Mr. Colpo was the inaccuracy of the death certificates that ultimately records the cause of death.[29,30] If these numbers are not accurate, then how can the studies be valid?

A good comprehensive (and more objective) source is the book *The Cholesterol Myths,* by Uffe Ravnskov MD [31], this is a very comprehensive look at how blaming cholesterol for heart disease is based on flimsy research, disappearing information and outright misrepresentation of facts. The most recent book I have read regarding the cholesterol lie is *The Great Cholesterol Myth* by Dr. Johnny Bowden and Stephen Sinatra

MD.[32] This book is a very good all-around look at the politics, the true indicators of heart disease (actually supported by the research), and the overall cholesterol lie that we have been led to believe.

Any of these books will open your eyes to the power and the political influence of the drug lobby, the edible oils industry, and the pharmaceutical industry. There seems to be a revolving door of employment between governmental agencies and people who work at the upper level of the drug companies.[33,34] Would it be too bold to suggest potential cronyism here?

The DVD version of The Oiling of America, by Mary Enig and Sally Fallon can be purchased online and is a video that I show during my REGENESIS lectures. This is a great presentation as it traces the origin of the problem back to the late 1800's. It gives a comprehensive view of how this all came about especially the politics and manipulation of the facts. It will be hard to get to the truth from your doctors as they are towing the orthodox line on this. If they don't practice within certain guidelines, they are ostracized by their peers or governing groups, as everyone must be on board. If doctors are not on board, they may find themselves practicing "outside of the box".

Statin drugs used in "treating" cholesterol, have more side effects to them than almost any other commonly prescribed drug I know of. They are highly profitable and are distributed widely in the American population as cholesterophobia spreads. One little fact that never seems to be mentioned in the cholesterol discussion is that the death rate goes up as cholesterol levels go below a certain point.[35] Low cholesterol levels are potentially associated with shorter life-spans due to increased incidence of cancers, depression, suicide, and diabetes.[36,37,38] I'll bet you didn't see that on TV in the Lipitor and Crestor commercials. What you did see, if you were paying attention, is that the disclaimers took more time than the sales pitch! For most people, there is little to no proof that taking statin drugs increases lifespan by one minute.

Low cholesterol levels are potentially associated with shorter life-spans due to increased incidence of cancers, depression, suicide, and diabetes.

I know a lot of people who were injured by statin drugs, some of them permanently. My cousin almost died from them and took two years to get over the damage that was done to her. Despite this, her doctor still wants her to take them. Unbelievable! Her doctor has even tried to go the back door route and encouraged her to take Red Rice Yeast extract. He is obviously on board with the orthodox line, and the prudent diet. As well intentioned as he is, he has been told the lie so many times, he believes it 100%.

A recent study conducted at Rochester Methodist Hospital, Mayo Clinic in Minnesota concluded that statin drug use increased the incidence of type two diabetes by 71% in post-menopausal women averaging 63 years of age.(39) Where was the news media on this one? A lot of money (billions) is spent on TV networks for drug advertising. I don't suspect that had anything to do with it.

There is a push now to test our children and if they fit the criteria, put them on statin drugs too. (40) We have lost our collective minds here. When are we going to stop the insanity and realize that our diets are killing us and now our children too? The emphasis here should be on diet, not on prescribing these toxic drugs to our precious children. Where are the "diet dictocrats" on this one? Given the increased incidence of diabetes in post-menopausal women and the countless side effects of these drugs, do we really want to expose our children to statins?

There is also talk of reducing the threshold of the lipid profile numbers at which statin drugs are prescribed. (41) I have a better idea. <u>How about teaching our parents and children about the importance of consuming quality fats and reducing inflammatory foods</u>? I have an idea that may be even better than that. LET'S TEACH OUR HEALTHCARE PROVIDERS THE TRUTH! This cholesterophobia problem is perpetuated by politics, fear-mongering, greed, and ignorance in a disconnected society.

According to *The Centers for Disease Control and Prevention*, medical costs for treating heart disease in 2010, was 444 billion dollars. (42) I can't help but think that if the same amount of money would have been spent on true prevention through correct dietary advice, we would not be dying of heart disease at the rate we see today in America. Our diets are killing us! I beg of you to do some reading and research on the subject. Be proactive in your health.

When I advise patients on diet and nutrition, they don't believe me at first and I get what I call "the look". I tell them to eat free range eggs every day and to use good quality fats including butter, coconut oil, and lard. I allow them to eat red meat and pork (providing that it is free range and grass fed). I tell them to eat bone in baked chicken and they are to eat the skin. All non-starchy vegetables are allowed. I also instruct them, as you have read in the water chapter, to consume ½ their body weight in ounces of water every day and to give up all of their man made beverages.

These recommendations are contrary to conventional wisdom. After a month or so, if they are following my program, most patients notice their blood tests are much improved. Cholesterol ratios, triglyceride levels, fasting sugars, A1C tests also improve. They are usually a few pounds lighter too. Their doctors just scratch their heads. How can this be? It's simple. Again, it's the use of processed foods, sugars, wheat products, rancid fats, stress, and smoking that create inflammation. These factors are what cause the cholesterol numbers to be "abnormal", not the ingestion of <u>quality cholesterol</u> and <u>quality fat</u> containing foods. (43)

Recently a friend of mine brought in a "dietary handout" he was given at his heart doctor's office. It was the prudent diet. The pamphlet was produced by Bell Institute of Health and Nutrition (General Mills), a

Honey Nut Cheerios logo was on the pamphlet. Of course at the top of the list of recommended foods were the "healthy grains" including Berry Burst Cheerios, biscuits made with Heart Smart Bisquick, breads, Cheerios, Doughnut-raised glazed, Honey Nut Cheerios, and MultiGrain Cheerios. The pamphlet suggested avoiding or limiting foods with tropical oils such as palm kernel and coconut oils. The recommendations were to replace saturated fats like butter and shortening, with liquid vegetable oils or trans-fat free soft margarine.[44] So it is still the same old song: low fat, high carbs (grains), and little to no quality saturated fats. Nothing is changing in spite of the fact that the research does not substantiate the diet-heart hypothesis that "quality" saturated fats cause heart disease.[45] The problems with the grains, especially wheat and its connection to inflammation (one of the major causes of poor health) were discussed at length in chapter 3.

Doctors still recommend the "prudent diet" that was promoted by the edible oil industry and others in the food industry that vilify natural saturated fats (their competition). This diet is low in cholesterol, grain based, fat free or reduced fat foods. Saturated fats are very limited and replaced mainly by man-made oils that are polyunsaturated also known as polyunsaturated fatty acids (PUFA's) . This diet was and is basically supported by the USDA's food pyramid and to some degree the new "Harvard Food Plate". It is still the "prudent diet" with a just a little different face on it. Look around, how is that working? It seems the more we adhere to the "prudent diet" including its six to eleven servings of grains per day, the sicker we are individually and as a country.

It seems the more we adhere to the "prudent diet", including its six to eleven servings of grains per day, the sicker we are...

Despite eating all of this low cholesterol or no cholesterol food, we sure do take a lot of cholesterol lowering drugs. We didn't do that when we were eating quality saturated fats at the turn of the twentieth century. Heart disease and cancers were not the pervasive diseases they are today. It is the man made processed foods and chemical additives in our food supply that cause most of our diseases. Why is this so hard for people to see?

> One of my patients, also a close friend of mine, recently came to me suffering from sciatica and bilateral knee pain so bad he was using crutches. He could not work and he could not go fishing, one of his favorite things to do in life. He had been to doctors regarding his knees and was told they were just wearing out. He was 305 lbs., a big guy to start with, and definitely too heavy for his frame. He will admit to you that he certainly did not eat very healthily. His job requires that he spend a lot of time traveling and he ate a lot of junk foods. His triglycerides were 355, his fasting sugars were 129, and his blood pressure was creeping upwards. After four months on my REGENESIS program, and some gentle, non-invasive lumbar decompression therapy for his sciatica, he is virtually pain free, his knees are much improved, and he is 60 lbs. lighter and counting.
>
> He went back to his medical doctor and had his yearly blood work done. The results in comparison to his last years tests were striking. His triglycerides were 45, his fasting blood sugar was 100 (still a little high but improving), his blood pressure was normal and his cholesterol ratios were perfect. His doctor asked him what he was doing and he told him about the diet and the vitamin program that I had him on. His doctor willingly approved of the great improvements in his health and told him that vitamins and minerals were the key to good health. This patient has been seeing this doctor for many years. If vitamins and minerals are the key to good health, why were they never recommended to him?

> I took the time to explain very carefully how he had to change his eating habits. I went into great detail regarding his supplement regimen and the care plan for his back and sciatica problem. I also made it perfectly clear that if he didn't take off the weight, his general health, and his knee and back problems would just get worse. He has been following the REGENESIS program to the letter. These remarkable results take time and can't be done in the 5 minutes that most doctors spend with patients these days. Health is a process, not an event.

Health is a process, not an event.

<u>Quality</u> fats have been unjustly, but successfully vilified by the edible oil industry. Our doctors and hospitals (the ones that provide and profit from soft drinks and provide chlorinated tap water to sick and dehydrated patients) are all on board too. I see doctors in my community eating margarine, "heart healthy" spreads and drinking diet sodas. I see the dietary recommendations handed to my patients by medical doctors and dietitians on pre-printed sheets it is always the "prudent diet" or the Mediterranean diet that recommends unhealthy man-made polyunsaturated fats and restriction of <u>quality</u> saturated fats.

On countless occasions while staying with my severely diabetic mother in the hospital, I saw tray after tray of white flour products, diet drinks, artificial sweeteners, hydrogenated oil based coffee creamers, and margarine spreads brought for her to eat. I don't know how anyone can blame heart attacks on butter and lard. It is so hard to find these things in the midst of all the hydrogenated margarines and imitation butter products on grocery store shelves, in hospitals and our public schools in this country. These so called "healthy heart spreads" are man-made of potentially rancid, highly processed, hydrogenated oils. I suspect that highly processed and hydrogenated fats are more responsible for our poor health because far more people consume these products than butter, coconut oil, or lard.

The French eat a lot more fat and cream than almost any other culture, yet they are far ahead of the US in longevity, this is called the French paradox. How can the French eat so much fat and drink so much wine and still have less heart related deaths than we do? The French consume quality fats and butter. They drink wine that contains resveratrol, a powerful antioxidant that can actually protect your organs and the lining of your arteries. Quality cholesterol is a powerful antioxidant that may also protect you against cancer.[46] Do they really consider this a paradox? Do they need to do some research? Maybe just a common sense look at it would suffice. I think a French chef would rather commit suicide than to cook something in margarine and skim milk as opposed to sweet cream and butter.

The REGENESIS program requires avoiding all hydrogenated fats, anything that contains trans-fats, all vegetable oils, and all foods that are fried in these bad fats! Don't eat potato chips, bloomin' onions, French fries, cellophane wrapped snack cakes, or donuts. If you read labels, you will find partially hydrogenated and trans-fats in thousands of packaged foods.

If you want to fry eggs, you can use butter. Fry them over low heat and over easy. The preferred method of cooking eggs is poached or soft boiled. If you place a fertilized egg in a warm environment, in 21 days it will produce a living breathing fully functional animal! A free range egg is a powerful food that is rich in life giving nutrients including quality cholesterol, proteins, vitamins, minerals and fatty acids. Do not be afraid of eggs, they too have been falsely vilified by the so called "experts". Just a side note here, eggs are nature's Viagra. Eating eggs increases oxygenation, largely due to their sulfur content. There is also high quality cholesterol in eggs. Remember that sex hormones have a very high cholesterol content.

Our brain is 2 % of our body weight but contains 25% of the body's cholesterol. Trillions of our cells are wrapped in fat. Think about this, we omit cholesterol rich eggs and quality saturated fats from our diet, (doctor's orders), then we're instructed to eat a low fat diet and replace those calories with grains and carbohydrates (refined and natural). We complicate this even more by following doctor's orders to take cholesterol lowering drugs.

So, we deplete our body of quality essential cholesterol, we further enhance that with a statin drug. How on earth do we expect our cholesterol rich cells (like neurons) to repair and maintain themselves? How can our very important cell walls function properly? We have to take erectile dysfunction (ED) drugs like the little blue pill.[47] We end up sitting in the separate Cialis bathtubs (explain that commercial to me, as I would want to be in the same tub). Our televisions are loaded with low testosterone (low-"T") commercials and consequently, low T drug lawsuits. A host of various diabetic medicines and treatments are added to this mess. Later in life we can't remember anything (Alzheimer's disease). It all sounds very profitable to me as cholesterol medicines, ED pills, testosterone replacement products, and Alzheimer's medicines are very expensive and profitable. Am I the only one that sees this insanity? Go ahead and call me a conspiracy theorist!

Look for a new and emerging term for diabetes, high cholesterol and decreasing cognition- "Type 3 diabetes".[48] This is thought to be the precursor to Alzheimer's disease. From a subjective point of view, it all seems to be man-made, or at least man induced. I personally think Alzheimer's is largely a man-made disease. Created from decades of promoting man-made polyunsaturated fats to replace natural saturated fats, pushing excessive servings of grains with the USDA food pyramid, the lie that is artificial sweeteners, our obsession/addiction to sugar, and the final nail, statin drugs.[49] This is a lethal long term combination. Cases of Alzheimer's disease are increasing exponentially in comparison to other diseases that affect older patients. Read the book *Grain Brain*, by Dr. David Perlmutter, it's a hard hitting look at this emerging phenomenon. The information in this book should really tic you off. Personally, I am already ticked off after watching my mother suffer for many years and eventually die from diabetes and its complications, coupled with poor medical advice. *Grain Brain* is very high on my must read list! It exposes the fallacy of years of bad advice given to diabetics by doctors and so called nutritionists.

If you cook free range grass fed beef, save the oil drippings from that in an air tight container. Quality lard is okay to use for cooking if you can find it, use it sparingly (I have a link to a quality lard product at *regenesis4health.com*). I suggest using olive oil for salad dressings only. If you insist on cooking with olive oil, do not cook on high heat, as it turns rancid very quickly when subjected to high heat. Working toward avoiding all man-made mass produced vegetable and seed oils is my highest recommendation.

Olive oil and coconut oil are two oils that I will allow on the program. What makes them different from corn oil, vegetable oils, and other edible oils, is the way they are made. They are not processed like the seed and corn based oils. All oils, even olive and coconut oil, will go rancid when exposed to heat or oxygen over time. If you use these oils, buy them in small bottles and store them properly and use them in a reasonable time frame. All oils can go rancid over time with exposure to light and or heat, olive oil and coconut oil are no exception.

Remember, I am not an advocate of eating fried foods. If you insist on eating fried foods I advise you to never eat over cooked, burned, or seared meats. You are far better off eating steamed or raw non-starchy vegetables and minimize or completely eliminate fried food consumption. I prefer that you bake, broil, or stew your meats. Use quality cuts of free range meats and grass fed red meats. Wild meats like venison and turkey are also a very good source of quality protein. These meats are naturally free range and are rich in omega 3 fats. Buffalo meat is also a favorite of mine if you know for sure it is free range and grass fed. Meat portions should be about the size of the palm of your hand.

I get a lot of argument over breakfast meats like bacon and sausage. I have given in a little here by allowing free range nitrite/nitrate free meats to be fried in their own fats and used so long as they are not burned during preparation, the same applies for steak. Eggs cooked in butter along with quality breakfast meats can be the highest protein and fat meal of the day. Be aware that most commercial sausage products contain MSG. I recommend not eating any more fried foods the rest of the day if you insist on starting your day with fried foods. As far as breakfast is concerned, cooking things like bacon in a toaster oven (broiled) and eating poached eggs would be preferred over cereals, pancakes, waffles, bagels, etc. Learn how to cook smart. Knock the dust off the old crock pot and use it often.

When red meat producing animals are fed grains, the omega 3 content is largely replaced by omega 6 fats.[50] One of the problems with the Standard American Diet (SAD) is the imbalance of omega 3 to omega 6 fats. When food is advertised as "grain fed", put it back. Americans consume far too much poor quality omega 6 fat. This is why I always recommend free range, grass fed beef, venison, or bison that is naturally rich in omega 3 fat.

I get questions about cholesterol almost daily in my office. While I am no expert, I have read extensively on the subject and I feel that the most important number on the lipid profile is the (non-fasting) triglyceride content.[51] The next most important number is the small particle low density lipoprotein (LDL) content; these two numbers are intimately related. For a more comprehensive explanation of this, Dr. William Davis, a preventative cardiologist, explains lipids and cholesterol very well in his book *Wheat Belly* [52] Again, the book *The Great Cholesterol Myth* by Dr. Johnny Bowden and cardiologist Dr. Stephen Sinatra does a great job of explaining the truth about cholesterol.

One of the goals of the REGENESIS program is to keep the triglyceride number under control by keeping insulin levels under control. This is done by keeping blood sugar levels low through avoidance of wheat, sugars, and starchy carbohydrates. Are you seeing a trend here? This is a repeating theme for a reason.

All of this must be done in conjunction with the use of quality natural fats and proper hydration. In almost all cases, when the triglycerides are low, the small particle LDL levels are low. The REGENESIS program will help to normalize total cholesterol levels, cholesterol ratios, and triglycerides in most people. This does not occur because I am a genius, it occurs because this program removes inflammatory foods and chemicals. INFLAMMATION IS THE PROBLEM! If you have followed the program and blood lipids are still off, it is most likely due to stress or smoking. You must reduce stress where you can, and if you are smoking in spite of the mountain of evidence regarding the dangers of smoking, find a way to STOP SMOKING!

The numbers on the lipid profile do mean something, I don't question that, it is the basic evaluation and then the treatment that I have the problem with. When a high saturated fat diet is combined with a highly processed carbohydrate diet, blood lipids elevate and ratios get out of kilter. It's always the fat that gets the blame; it's actually the sugar and the wheat that's the problem. If you are eating quality saturated fats along with healthy vegetables and you are avoiding all of the other health land mines, your cholesterol should be "normal". I have helped a lot of people attain this with diet alone. The intake of <u>quality dietary fats</u> has little to no effect on the elevation of cholesterol numbers.[53] It is the intake of excessive carbohydrates, junk food, wheat products, food additives, smoking, and stress that cause cholesterol numbers to become altered because they create inflammation. I will continue to make this point over and over (yes I know it is redundant).

Dr. Stephen Sinatra a cardiologist and author of *The Great Cholesterol Myth*, says that lowering cholesterol has little to nothing to do with lowering the risk of heart disease.[54] This takes a lot of courage to stand up against the tidal wave of misinformation generated by his peers, the scientific community and the media.

If you really want to get specific tests for heart disease, have your C-reactive protein, lipoprotein-a, and homocysteine levels checked. If these numbers are high in combination with high non-fasting or fasting triglycerides, severely elevated cholesterol numbers, and abnormal cholesterol ratios, and a big ol'belly, you could have stroke or a potential heart problem brewing. The REGENESIS program has helped many of my patients bring these values (and their big ol' bellies) back into normal and healthy ranges. A quality diet with all the essential nutrients including quality saturated fats, antioxidants, pure water, and no food chemicals, supports healthy cholesterol and triglyceride levels.

If you follow the program for a few weeks and are concerned about eating fats and eggs, ask your doctor to order a lipid profile. There are also online blood testing companies if you do not have a doctor. The tests are inexpensive and will give you some peace of mind if you suffer from cholesterophobia. If your numbers are not yet in balance, it could be your stress levels, or you may not have eliminated all of your sugars, wheat products, soft drinks, and junk foods. If you smoke, stop or you will never attain good health (there is that repeating theme again). If you continue to have elevated lipid profiles in spite of making significant changes, you could have familial hypercholesterolemia, this should be managed by your doctor. Remember you must drink adequate amounts of water on the program!

If you smoke, stop or you will never attain good health.

Supplementing your diet with eicosapentaenoic acid/ docosahexaenoic acid (EPA/DHA), most commonly found in cold water fish oils, insures that you are getting enough of the essential fatty acids in the proper ratio. Remember, the Standard American Diet is far too heavy in poor quality omega 6 oils and not enough omega 3 oils. Hemp oil is very well balanced in this regard. Most EPA/DHA comes from cold water ocean fish. Some people do not like the taste or the after taste of fish oils. Hemp and flax seed oils are good alternatives for some people. Eating quality wild caught fish is a good way to get quality essential fatty acids. Salmon, sardine, and Krill are the best sources of EPA/DHA. These oils are essential to brain structure and function, heart health, hormone production, and cognition as well as countless other body functions. Essential oils are crucial for good health and make-up the outer most part of your cells (cell walls).

Nuts and seeds are a good food source and are nutrient dense. I always recommend organic if possible. Nuts contain phytates that can interfere with absorption of minerals. Soaking nuts greatly reduces their phytic acid content. Soaked or sprouted organic nuts are the most desirable. They can be hard to find, but are worth the hunt. High on my list of recommendations is almonds, walnuts, pistachios, and pecans. Nuts are great to snack on if you get hungry between meals. They do contain some carbohydrates and should be used sparingly. Eight to ten nuts is usually the right amount to use between meals. Organic nuts contain healthy oils. Walnut oils are particularly good for killing parasites. Almonds and apricot seeds have natural anti-cancer properties due to the B-17 (laetrile) content. I purchase sprouted or soaked organic nuts and nut butters from Blue Mountain Organics. I have a link to their website at *regenesis4health.com*.

Nut butters like almond butter are allowed on the REGENESIS program. Peanut butter is not allowed, as peanuts are not nuts, they are beans and contain phytates that hamper mineral absorption, as well as aflatoxins that are cancer causing chemicals produced by two different molds commonly found on peanuts.

This is a good place to do a summary. You should be drinking adequate amounts of pure water, working on being wheat free, and eliminating the sugars and sugar substitutes from your diet. Looking for all of the bad fats in your cupboards and beginning to think differently about how you prepare foods. Learn how to use a crock pot and how to poach eggs.

6

Food Additives

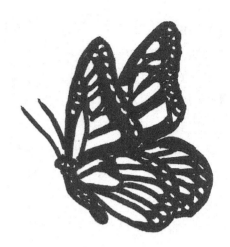

"A Who's Who of pesticides is therefore of concern to us all. If we are going to live so intimately with these chemicals eating and drinking them, taking them into the very marrow of our bones – we had better know something about their nature and their power."
Rachel Carson, Silent Spring

THIS IS AN extensive topic so I just want to zero in on a few food additives that are common in our food supply. Food additives are used for color, preservation, texture, and flavor enhancement. There are thousands of chemicals in manufactured foods, some are much worse than others. It is the accumulated effect of these chemicals that I am concerned about. There are carcinogens, allergens, toxins, hormone disrupters, and even behavioral disrupters in our national food supply. All of the additives in this chapter are allowed by the FDA. Do not rely on the FDA or the food industry in general to adequately inform or protect you.

MSG

Number one on the radar is monosodium glutamate (MSG), aka free glutamic acid. This additive is used mainly as a flavor enhancer. It does many things, including destroying nerve cells. Under certain conditions

MSG can cross the blood brain barrier (a selective barrier that protects the central nervous system). These conditions include: head injury, hypertension, elevated core temperature, viral or bacterial infections of the brain and spinal cord, and exposure to heavy metals. Once inside the blood brain barrier, MSG can literally excite neurons to death. This type of toxin is called an excitotoxin. I highly recommend the book *Excitotoxins The Taste that Kills*[1], by Dr. Russell Blaylock a neurosurgeon who has studied the neurological effects of Aspartame and MSG. His book goes into great detail about the harmful effects of these and other additives on our health and the health of our children.

MSG was first introduced as "Accent", a flavor enhancing agent. There are forty different products that do not mention MSG, but contain MSG in them because food producers know that people are looking for it on food labels. Some of the food additives that contain MSG are calcium caseinate, autolyzed yeast, hydrolyzed protein, yeast food, textured protein, glutamic acid, natural flavor, and others. The labeling laws do not require some of these food products that contain MSG or free glutamic acid to be listed as individual ingredients. As a result, free glutamic acid is in a lot of foods that are not mentioned on the label.

MSG is highly suspected in causing "Chinese Restaurant Syndrome" also known as "MSG Symptom Complex". Symptoms include rapid heartbeat, headache, chest pain, numbness and burning around the mouth, sweating, flushing, and a sense of facial pressure or swelling. It has also been linked as a possible cause of nausea, depression, eye damage, slurred speech, fatigue, drowsiness, and hives, and this is the short list. MSG has been potentially linked to neurological diseases like Parkinson's, Huntington's disease, Lou Gehrig's disease and Alzheimer's [2]. What an impressive list by this FDA approved food additive! It is found in canned soups, yogurt, potato chips and other crunchy snack foods, TV dinners, boxed pizzas, sauces used in restaurants, boullion and almost anything with a "flavor packet". Obviously, it's common in our food supply! Eliminating MSG from your diet is a crucial step in recovering your health.

Hydrolyzed protein

Hydrolyzed proteins are an interesting taste enhancing food additive and particularly dangerous, possibly more ominous than MSG. It is a process where proteins from corn, whey, soy, and wheat, are separated by water (hydrolysis), then completed by a chemical process. This chemical process requires hydrochloric acid, then sodium hydroxide as a neutralizing agent. Does this sound like something natural? This separation yields a brown sludge that is allowed to dry into a powder and is particularly salty to the taste. The end product contains free glutamic acid, the same glutamic acid found in MSG. It also contains cystoic acid and aspartate, two more excitotoxins. It has been linked to the same neurological diseases as MSG but it is a suspected carcinogen making it potentially more dangerous than MSG. These products are used in a lot of foods including imitation meat products, and various meats like barbecue for seasoning. This seasoning can be found in a lot of canned foods and is often used instead of MSG because of the loophole in labeling. This loophole allows certain food additives that may contain anywhere from twenty to sixty percent MSG to be called "natural flavoring".[3] It seems to me that if things were "natural" you would proudly list what it is on the label. You can see "natural flavoring" on thousands of products on your grocery store shelves. "Natural flavorings" are in a lot of the products that you and your children eat every day if you eat processed canned foods or frozen foods like TV dinners.

Children are five times more sensitive to these dangerous neruotoxins than adults. It has also been discovered that humans are many times more sensitive to MSG and hydrolyzed proteins than rats or other experimental animals like chimpanzees.[4] The industry deliberately did experimentation on animals that are not as sensitive as humans to MSG.

Don't count on the food industry or governmental agencies to protect you! Again, your health is your responsibility.

Bisphenol-A (BPA)

Another chemical that is found in food is Bisphenol-A, this is one of the highest volume produced chemicals in the world.[5] Technically, BPA is not a food additive but ends up in our foods because it is used in can liners, plastic bottles, storage containers, and water pipes. It is also found on cash register receipts. So if your job involves handling cash register receipts, I would highly recommend wearing some form of protective glove (like a surgical rubber or latex glove) at work.

BPA has been linked to hyperactivity, learning disabilities, structural brain damage, obesity, altered immune function, early puberty, ovarian dysfunction, prostate cancer, enlarged prostate, liver damage, and heart disease. There is evidence that BPA accumulates in human tissues including breast milk. [6]

If you remember in the chapter on water, I suggested you use a glass container to carry your filtered water in. BPA in plastic water bottles is one of the main reasons not to purchase and use bottled water. The FDA says BPA is safe.

There are only a few companies that use BPA free food cans, another one of many reasons to cook foods at home from fresh ingredients. BPA was the subject of a lot of media coverage. The discussion in the mainstream media regarding BPA went away very quickly. This is very suspicious to me.

Nitrites and Nitrates

Nitrites and nitrates are substances found in processed meats like bacon, sausage, deli meats, hot dogs, bologna, potted meats, and canned meats. They are also found in celery and other vegetables naturally. They serve as color stabilizers and as preservatives. The problem with nitrites and nitrates is that they produce nitrosamines when exposed to high heat. Nitrosamine is strongly linked to gastric cancer, colon cancer, pancreatic cancer and chronic obstructive pulmonary disease COPD.[7] This is why I am always harping on not eating burned or seared meats. It is virtually impossible to avoid nitrites and nitrates, but it is possible not to burn your meats during the cooking process. Baking, broiling, and stewing meats are the preferable means of preparation. Purchasing sodium nitrite and sodium nitrate free meats significantly reduces exposure to these potential toxic food additives.

Brominated Vegetable Oil (BVO)

Brominated Vegetable Oil is a flame retardant and a clouding agent that has been banned from foods in Japan, India and throughout Europe. It is most commonly found in soft drinks in America. About 10% of soft drinks contain BVO. It is most commonly found in Mountain Dew, Fresca original citrus, Sunkist Pineapple, Powerade Strawberry Lemonade, Fanta Orange, Squirt [8] and various copy-cat sodas purchased at big box stores with their own brand names. Coca-cola and Pepsico are slowly replacing BVO in their beverages with esterified rosin.

Bromine is an endocrine disruptor, it interferes with your body's ability to adequately hold and use iodine which is crucial for proper thyroid function. Bromine can cause skin rashes, severe acne, fatigue, cardiac arrhythmia, acute paranoid schizophrenia, and other mental disorders [9] This is a most impressive list for a product that most Americans have never heard of. I see a lot of our teenagers with severe acne drinking soft drinks and so called "power drinks" that contain BVO. These drinks along with the excessive consumption of wheat products and sugars are a recipe for acne, obesity, and a host of other maladies.

You see highly paid athletes on TV drinking Gatorade and the winning coach gets the Gatorade bath at the end of the game, no wonder our kids think it is good for them. Oh, by the way, Gatorade, Powerade, and other commercial sports drinks only contain two minerals, sodium and potassium.

Athletes need sixty or more minerals to replace the minerals used up in high performance sports. There was a recent commercial showing a high intensity athlete with enhanced green and blue sweat coming out of his sweat pores. To me that is exactly what it should look like, green and blue food colorings and brominated vegetable oils coming out thru the sweat glands. Athletes need way more than two minerals, sugar, unnatural oils, and food colorants to perform at a high level for extended periods of time.

A recent online petition initiated by a high school sophomore created a heightened awareness of BVO in popular soft drinks and sports drinks, in particular Gatorade. This petition has been said to have prompted Pepsico, the manufacturer of Gatorade, to remove BVO from its drinks in America. PepsiCo denies that it removed BVO from Gatorade because of the petition.[10] As of the writing of this book, Pepsico has removed BVO from Gatorade, but not from one of their most popular soft drinks, Mountain Dew. Other drink manufacturing companies are still using this additive. At least Pepsico stepped up and did the right thing in their Gatorade products. BVO is slowly starting to be replaced with esterified rosins in sports drinks and soft drinks as public awareness increases. For what it's worth, BVO is deemed safe by the FDA.

Sugar Substitutes

One of the most difficult things to do in changing your lifestyle is giving up processed sugar. This becomes very obvious when the headaches start about 2 or 3 days after one stops consuming sugars. We start looking for something acceptable to replace sugar with. Unfortunately for the consumer, there is a lot of misinformation about sugar substitutes regarding their safety and actual effects on human health. This is a very broad and difficult topic to cover in an introductory self-help book. I will provide several resources in the pages that follow if more information is desired. It is very important that you become familiar with these products and the foods that contain them.

Aspartame

The most widely used artificial sweetener is Aspartame, now called Amino Sweet. Other aspartame products include Nutra-Sweet, Equal, and Canderel. Aspartame has been the source of much controversy. This product was introduced by G.D. Searle & Co. in late 1979 and early 1980. It is now one of the most widely used sugar substitutes in America. Diabetics use a lot of this sweetener. Aspartame is 200 times sweeter than sugar and has a slight after-taste.(11) The manufacturer claims that Aspartame is made from nature. While it is true that the ingredients in Aspartame are found in nature, the process by which it is made is chemical, not natural. Again the story of Aspartame is very well described by Dr. Russell Blaylock, MD. in *Excitotoxins: The Taste that Kills*. These chemicals have the potential to cross the blood brain barrier and are suspected in contributing to neurological diseases. Aspartame also crosses through the placenta, which connects a developing fetus to the uterine wall. If an expectant mother eats MSG or Aspartame, or most any other chemical for that matter, it is a good possibility it will cross the placental barrier into the sensitive nerve tissues of the developing child. (12)

Aspartame was approved by the FDA for use in all foods in 1996. It is currently found in over 6000 food products worldwide. One of the primary ingredients in Aspartame is the amino acid phenylalanine. This substance should be avoided by people with a condition called Phenylketonuria. When Aspartame breaks down after consumption, it changes into Phenylalanine, Aspartic Acid, and Methanol (a deadly metabolic poison that cannot be digested). These agents can break down further into formic acid (used to kill ants) and formaldehyde (embalming fluid).(13) So if you are okay with an ant killing metabolic poison mixed with embalming fluids floating around in your body, then keep using your diet drinks and sugar free treats that contain Aspartame. If you really want to get some insight on Aspartame, I highly recommend the book *The Deadly Deception,* by Mary Nash Stoddard.(14) This book was published in 1998, so the information is far from new. She exposes the power of politics and large corporations, as well as the insidious dangers of consuming Aspartame. Once you've read it, you will have no doubts to the dangers of this food additive. This is a must read. Although many studies have been done, controversy over this sweetener rages on.

One of the many reasons that I don't allow Aspartame on my program is that I generally do not trust research that has been done, or paid for, by parties that have something to gain from the outcome of the research. I have taken many patients off of Aspartame and they always have marked improvement. After being on the REGENESIS program for a while, many vegetables like carrots or celery become very sweet tasting. I want you to partake in nature's foods as you were meant to and move away from all processed foods. The following two lists contain conditions that can be caused by, mimicked by, or triggered by Aspartame (15):

Headaches	Nausea	Vertigo	Personality changes	Blindness
Hearing Loss	Tinnitus	Insomnia	Anxiety	Hyperactivity
Numbness	Fatigue	Skin lesions	Blurred vision	Muscle Cramps
Memory Loss	Joint pain	Depression	Slurred speech	Arrythmias
Chest Pain	Edema	PMS	Mood changes	Increased appetite

Aspartame may trigger or mimic the following illnesses:

Chronic Fatigue Syndrome	Epstein-Barr	Post-Polio syndrome
Lyme's Disease	Menieres' Disease	Alzheimer' Disease
ALS (Lou Gehrig's)	Epilepsy	Multiple Sclerosis
Hypothyroidism	Increased sensitivity from mercury amalgam fillings	

A new study from Harvard links Aspartame to blood cancers. The research revealed that when men consumed one or more sodas sweetened with aspartame, there was an increase in Non-Hodgkin's Lymphoma and multiple myeloma. There was an increase in Leukemia when the sample of men and women were combined in the study.(16) The study has been criticized by many, but it does makes a strong suggestion in my mind that Aspartame should be eliminated. Where were these research critics when the Vioxx studies were done? I don't want to wait for the next "study", I have enough doubt already from other sources on the dangers of Aspartame. How much more research needs to be done before we wake up? Again, I see local doctors consuming diet drinks; most of them don't understand it either. You can buy these diet drinks in hospitals that proudly display the picture of the hospital on the front of the vending machines! As I have mentioned previously, the hospitals share the profits from the sale of these unhealthy products.

Splenda (aka Sucralose)

Sucralose (Splenda) is another sweetener that is widely used in our food supply. I think they call it Splenda because its chemical name is: 1-6-dichloro-1-6dideosy-BETA-D-fructofuranosyl-4-chloro-4-deoxy-alpha-D-galactopyranoside. That just rolls off the tongue doesn't it? They say it's made from nature, doesn't sound natural to me. Usage of Splenda is increasing approximately 10% per year in America. It's found in over 4000 food products. It's not as controversial as Aspartame, but there is mounting evidence that it has many side effects and compromises your health. The molecular structure of Splenda highly resembles DDT, an insecticide that was banned many years ago but can still be found in most water supplies around the world. To date, no long term study has been conducted on the potentially harmful effects of Splenda. As of 2009, the longest human study was four days. (17)

Splenda is composed of one sugar molecule with three chlorine molecules attached to it. This is done by a chemical process, which means Splenda is a processed chemical food additive. For that reason alone, I don't recommend its use. Splenda increases the pH of the intestines, reduces beneficial bacteria in the gut, and is absorbed by body fat. It has prompted a variety of consumer complaints like, gastrointestinal problems, migraine, seizures, weight gain, and skin rashes among others [18]. Again, nature will provide you with sweetness if you follow the plan. A good book to read about Sucralose is - *Splenda, Is It Safe Or Not,* by Dr. Janet Starr Hull. [19]

Agave

Everyone thought Agave (a cactus plant extract) was going to be the great savior of sweeteners, but it too has some problems. It's promoted as a natural sweetener taken from the Yucca plant. In reality, it is a highly refined chemically rendered sugar that is very similar to high fructose corn syrup. Use of Agave can contribute to triglyceride and obesity issues. It also mimics most, if not all, of the problems caused by high fructose corn syrup. [20] It must be avoided and is not recommended on the REGENESIS program

Sugar Alcohols

Sugar alcohols are another type of artificial sweetener used pervasively in the "sugar free" food industry. They are: Mannitol, Sorbitol, Xylitol, Lacitol, Maltitol, Erythritol, and Isomalt. These compounds contain a sugar on one end of the molecule and an alcohol on the other end. They are commonly found in chewing gum and toothpaste especially Xylitol and Sorbitol. At one time I allowed people on the plan to use Xylitol until I researched it a little more. Xylitol has been potentially implicated in causing tumors in some animal studies, therefore I have discontinued suggesting it even for short term use. It's just not worth the long term risk. Also worth noting is that Xylitol can be fatal to your pets. [21]

Acesulfame-K

Acesulfame-K (acesulfame potassium) is an artificial sweetener approved by the FDA in 1988 for use in dry beverage mixes, gelatin desserts, non-dairy creamers, instant coffee, teas, and candies. It has obviously been approved for use in soda as I have seen it on the labels of flavoring concentrates used in the home soda making appliances. The research has been scant and poorly done on this food additive. There is considerable evidence that it may be carcinogenic. In researching this chemical, I found some interesting quotes from very qualified doctors on the questionable research. Marvin Schneiderman, Ph.D and former Associate Director of Field Studies and Statistics at the National Cancer Institute said:

> *I find the actual studies and the data analysis seriously flawed. New tests, properly designed, executed, and analyzed are needed. The usual consequences of poor tests, is to make it harder to find any effects. Despite the low quality of the studies reported to you, I find that there is evidence of carcinogenicity.* (22)

This is no small comment from a very qualified individual, yet our friends and ardent protectors of Americans, the FDA, continues to allow Acesulfame-K to be used in the food supply. For some other qualified comments, go to the website, www.holisticmed.com/acek.

The Delaney Clause occurred in 1958 named after Congressman James Delaney of N.Y. It was an amendment to the Foods, Drugs and Cosmetic Act of 1938 (23). Its main purpose was to keep dangerous carcinogens like benzene, methanol and numerous other chemicals out of the food supply. After reading some of the legal mumbo junk, it seems that this amendment was targeted at food additives initially. The Delaney Clause has been used to challenge chemicals that are used in the production of food additives. Food colorings and sweeteners like Acesulfame K have been challenged under the Delaney Clause. The results of the hearings are a little disturbing and provide the ammo I need when I tell you that the food industry, government or the FDA is not going to adequately protect you. The following statement regarding Acesulfame K was made by the court from the Scott vs. FDA ruling from the United States Court of Appeals, Sixth Circuit. Argued on Jan 25, 1984 and decided on Feb. 23, 1984.

> The Delaney Clause applies to the additive itself and not to the constituents used to process the additive. Thus, where an additive has not been shown to cause cancer even though it contains a carcinogenic impurity, the additive is not subject to the legal effect of the Delaney Clause. Rather, the additive is properly evaluated under the general safety standard using risk assessment procedures to determine whether there is reasonable certainty that no harm will result from the proposed use of the additive. [Scott v. FDA, 728F.2d 322) 6th Cir. 1984)]. (24)

The first sentence in that clause says it all for me. So while the "jury is still out" when it comes to Acesulfame K, I highly recommend against its use. It is not allowed on the REGENESIS program.

Many of the artificial sweeteners stimulate the appetite; this is not useful if you are trying to lose weight and get healthy. Any benefit gained by the reduction in sugar calories is more than offset by potential toxicity and the increased stimulation of the appetite. Also, remember back to our discussion on how foods trigger genetic responses. I could only imagine what these artificial sweeteners signal to your genes. Let me point out here again that all of the so called "artificial sweeteners" have potential side effects.

If you have health problems, it doesn't make sense to add these chemicals to the already toxic situation that exists in your body. For a lot of people, giving up sugars and sweeteners is the hardest part of any get healthy program. Quality <u>pure stevia drops</u> remain the only valid choice of sweeteners for me. I want people to develop tastes for natural sugars found in whole organic foods. This concept is crucial to your long term success and health.

In the future, we will learn much more about these chemical sweeteners especially Aspartame, Sucralose, and Acesulfame-K. I believe what we'll discover will not be pretty. It is my opinion that there are no safe artificial sweeteners on the market. Americans have such a sweet tooth because of their excessive use of sugars and other sweeteners. They are constantly searching for sweet satisfaction.

It takes some time to appreciate Mother Nature's bounty after you have been consuming junk foods for years.

If you follow the REGENESIS program, and begin to use water as your primary beverage, this alone will help wean you from the need for sugary soft drinks. Once you have weaned yourself from sugar, you will appreciate how sweet nature's foods are. It takes some time to appreciate Mother Nature's bounty after you have been consuming junk foods for years. I have helped many patients realize that these artificial man made sweeteners are some of the worst chemicals you can put in your body. I personally feel they should have a skull and crossbones warning on them. To follow the REGENESIS program it's imperative that these chemicals are never used again in your lifetime. The REGENESIS program is designed to get you back as close to nature as possible. Chemicals made by man are not even close to nature in spite of how they are advertised.

Acrylamide

Acrylamide is a substance found in starchy (carbohydrate) foods that have been heated. Most notably potato chips, peanut butter, breads,

French fries, cereals, coffee, and popcorn (there are others). The discovery of acrylamide was made in 2002 by Swedish researchers. The EPA has classified acrylamide as a Group B2, probable carcinogen; acrylamide has been shown to cause cancer and neurotoxic effects in animal studies. (25)

Here again, another reason to avoid breads, cereals, and fried foods especially fried carbohydrates. All of the research I looked at suggested, of course, that more research is needed. I am not going to wait on the research to eliminate super-heated carbohydrates from the REGENESIS program, they are not allowed. If you follow the eating guidelines, your exposure to acrylamide will be minimal to zero.

Food Colorings

In an article titled "Food dyes: A Rainbow of Risks", the Center for Science in The Public Interest (CSPI), reported on studies that indicated a five-fold increase in the use of food dyes since 1955. Since food dyes are typically used in man-made processed foods, it's an alarming indicator of the increased consumption of processed foods in America. Red 40, Yellow 5, and Yellow 6 make up approximately 90% of all dyes used (26). These food colorings are still allowed in our food supply as well as body care products, medicines, and vitamin products. Most of these food dyes are made from a petroleum base.

In the 70's, a San Francisco doctor named Benjamin Feingold began taking his adult and child patients who had behavioral problems off of food dyes. His results were convincing. It did seem to prove a cause and effect relationship between behavioral problems and food dyes (27). Children in particular are 5 to 60 times (not percent, but times) more susceptible to the effects of carcinogens.(28) Studies on food dyes were done considering 1990 food dye consumption, that number is up more than 50% in essence making the research invalid for me. Look at all of the food colorings used in foods that are directly advertised to your children on TV. Read the labels!

Food dyes are studied individually. These isolated studies do not account for the possible toxic synergistic effects of dyes on each other, with other foods, or other environmental chemicals. According to the CSPI, food colorings can contain up to and in some cases more than ten percent impurities from the manufacturing process. (29)

Bound chemicals (ones that attach during the manufacturing process) are not typically evaluated when food dyes are studied. Bound benzidine has been found in Yellow 5 and 6 and is a known carcinogen. Other bound chemicals have been found in Red 40. (30)

Quoting again from the Scott v. FDA case of 1984 that also included challenges to the chemicals used in manufacturing food colorings:

> [T]he Agency does not believe that it is disregarding the Delaney Clause. In draft ing the Delaney Clause, Congress implicitly recognized that known carcinogens might be present in color additives as intermediaries or impurities but at levels too low to trigger a response in conventional test systems. Congress apparently concluded that the presence of these intermediaries or impurities at these low levels was acceptable. This legislative judgement accounts for the absence of any requirement in the Delaney Clause that the impurities and intermediaries in a color additive, rather than the additive as a whole, be tested or otherwise evaluated for safety. Thus, Congress drew a rough, quantitative dis- tinction between a color additive that is deemed unsafe under the Delaney Clause because it causes cancer, and an additive that is not subject to the Delaney Clause because it does not cause cancer even though one of its constituents does. FDA's decision on D&C Green No. 5 is consistent with this distinction. [Scott v. FDA, 728 F.2d 322(6th Cir. 1984)]. (31)

The last part of that ruling should prove to you that it's about legal interpretation, not your health! The bottom line here is that lawyers do what lawyers always do, they find the weaknesses in the system. The food industry always seems to find or create a crack that allows them to carry on business as usual so they can maximize profits. The result is that unsuspecting consumers and their children are still exposed to chemicals that are known carcinogens. The general thinking here is that the carcinogen is not in enough of a concentration to cause a "response". What about the "response" of decades of being exposed to a potential carcinogen from food additives? We consume a lot more food colorings now than in 1984 when this ruling was made. To me this is not worth it as food colorings add absolutely nothing of nutritional value.

Five of the most common food dyes are Red 40, Yellow 5 (Tartraine), Blue 2, Citrus red 2, and Yellow 6 (Sunset Yellow). These food dyes make up most of the food dyes used in many of the products we use every day. These dyes can cause a long list of problems:

Stomach Upset	ADHD	Headaches	Behavioral Issues
Anxiety	Hives	Itching	Heart Palpitations
Depression	Diarrhea	Vomiting	Blurred vision
Sleep Disturbances	Cancer [32]		

These colorants are found in our foods, vitamins, candies, cosmetics, cheese sauces, energy drinks, sodas, ice cream, jams, cake mixes and many other products. Food colorings are not necessary, they contribute nothing nutritionally. As usual, it always seems that these food chemicals "need more research". I don't know about you, but I don't need any more evidence. If you eat foods that are not processed or packaged, and take supplements that are not loaded with food colorants you can avoid these highly questionable chemicals.

Let's face it, we live in a chemical world but you can do a lot to limit your exposure to chemicals with some attention to your purchases. You must learn to read the food labels as these food colorings are in a lot of things that we consume. Eat the foods provided by nature and unprocessed by man's hand. The more processed a food is, the more likely it will contain chemicals along with the contaminants associated with production of those chemicals. Following the REGENESIS program helps to eliminate most, if not all, toxic food additives.

I could have written several chapters on food additives. The ones I went over here are some of the most common and most harmful. The thing I would like for you to take away here is that the food industry uses hundreds of chemicals in common every day foods that you purchase at your local grocery store. There is no way to know the potential cumulative effects of all these chemicals and the millions of combinations that they could create in our bodies. This is why I am so insistent that you cook as much as you can from scratch and avoid processed foods.

The fact is that if you follow the program, you won't have to concern yourself with food additives, lawyers and Supreme Court decisions, or the Delaney Clause, there won't be any food colorings in your diet or vitamins. You will be in charge, not the government, the FDA, or your doctor! You will be driving your own health bus, and hopefully your family and loved ones will be on board. There will not be MSG, Aspartame, BVO, BPA, sugar alcohols, food colorings, or other potentially harmful things in your foods. You can start to identify and eliminate as many man-made chemicals as you can from your environment. The next chapter introduces you to some of the problems that exist in your home other than in your food cupboards.

7

Chemical Madness

"Take care of your body, it's the only place you have to live."
Jim Rohn

IN ORDER TO recapture your health, it's important to understand that we are being exposed to hundreds if not thousands of chemicals every day. I want you to know why it is so important to identify areas that you can reduce your chemical exposure and then I want you to take the necessary steps to remove these toxic chemicals from your life. One hundred percent elimination is not possible.

Some of the chemicals are very obvious and some are hidden in our everyday products. Over 20 million synthetic chemicals have been created, somewhere between 50,000 and 100,000 synthetic chemicals are used in commerce (production of things we use), and 1 million new synthetic chemicals are created every year. These chemicals are organic and non-organic. The production of these chemicals began in the mid 1800's. The most potent of the organic variety called persistent organic pollutants (POP's) are the dioxins. The most famous of the dioxins is Agent Orange that was used over the jungles of Viet-Nam. It has harmed and killed so many of our Viet-Nam veterans. [1] I personally had a good friend that died from Agent Orange exposure in Viet Nam.

There is no way to know how the different combinations of these thousands of chemicals can harm us. These chemicals are found in our furniture, clothing, building products, foods, body care products and cosmetics. This doesn't even take into account air pollution, water pollution and medicines, that's right medicines are mostly chemicals. Traces of medicines are now being found in surface water runoff [2].

Chemicals are causing a lot of the diseases we are dying from in America and abroad, it is a global issue. Pesticides and herbicides have a strong connection to many of the cancers that kill us.[3] Over time things as simple as talcum powder and shampoos can have deadly toxic effects. Hair-spray, fingernail polish, hair dyes, body lotions are not exempt either, as the cosmetic industry is largely unregulated.

Jackie Kennedy Onassis died from non-Hodgkin's lymphoma. She endured caustic chemotherapy treatments for the disease.[4] There is some evidence this disease can be caused by hair dyes, particularly the darker ones, although this was never absolutely proven, hair dyes were very likely a contributing factor to her early death. Her personal hairdresser, Peter Lamas, has on his website- *"And then there was Jacqueline Kennedy Onassis, a client for whom I did hair and frequently applied hair die. Ms. Kennedy died too young from Non-Hodgkin's lymphoma cancer. Her doctors have stated publicly they believe her hair dye probably contributed to causing her death."* [5]

Many of these chemicals have a cumulative toxic potential over time.

Food additives, artificial sweeteners, food colorings and preservatives are pervasive in our food supply. Many of these chemicals have a cumulative toxic potential over time. Add this to the effects of other chemicals found in our environment and the toxic cumulative combinations are almost infinite and the potential for harm is huge.

There have been many good books written on the chemicals that are found in our environment. A good one to start with is *Toxic Beauty* by Samuel Epstien MD.(6) This book is about the cosmetic and body care industry and how over 200 toxic chemicals are allowed in our everyday body care products. These chemicals are potential carcinogens, skin irritants, endocrine disrupters, and neurotoxins. If you use modern cosmetics, this book is a must read. Dr. Epstien sounded the alarm on how chemicals were causing cancer in a hard hitting book *The Politics of Cancer.* (7) It is a scathing review of how nothing has been done to curb these chemicals from our lives. The book also calls out the medical profession, the FDA, and other agencies, for not doing their part to educate or warn the public in this most important health concern.

It's not my intention to delve into all of the minute details of this problem. What I hope to accomplish is to make you aware of the problem. You should educate yourself on the potential problems that are associated with chemical exposure. There are a lot of books and information on the web that will help you make good decisions. Removing or limiting your exposure to chemicals in your everyday life will greatly improve your overall health, function, and longevity.

Epstien's book *The Politics of Cancer,* clearly makes the point that we know what causes cancer, and that we have known this for years. His book was written in the 1980's. If we have known what causes cancer for years, why hasn't every citizen of the United States been sent notification? Why are these chemicals still allowed in our environment? Who is holding the chemical companies accountable? Where is the EPA with its regulations? Where are our doctors on this? Have they been made aware? If the doctors are aware, then why didn't we get a notice, or a warning, or an All Points Bulletin? If these chemicals cause cancers, why have they been allowed to permeate our lives to the degree they have? There should be skull and cross-bone warnings on our personal care products, hair colorings, some medicines (prescription and non-prescription), artificial sweeteners, talcum powder, air fresheners, mattresses, no iron shirts, paints, construction materials, and foods with chemicals in them. There should be warnings in our new cars about that "new car smell" which is the formaldehyde and other chemicals in the interior fabrics that can make us sick.

If you think the governmental agencies that should be protecting us are doing their jobs, you are not paying attention. The truth will be very well hidden because all of the emphasis for the harm done by these chemicals is placed on very expensive and very profitable treatments not prevention. A 2004 study published in the medical journal *Clinical Oncology* on chemotherapy as a treatment for malignant cancers, reveals that chemotherapy has a 97% (or better) failure rate over five years (8) and costs patients and their insurance providers thousands and thousands of dollars. Cancer is such a fearful thing and chemotherapy use is driven by desperation and fear on the patient's part, and very high profits for the drug and medical industry.

Oncologists are allowed to purchase their chemotherapy from drug companies and then mark it up to the patients and their insurance companies. This is called "buy and bill". The typical mark up for doctors is about 6%. That is not a large mark-up unless you are talking about a five or ten thousand dollar drug or infusion (6% of 10,000 dollars is 600 dollars). No other doctors are allowed to do this except for some neurologists that use infusions for Multiple Sclerosis treatments. There's no wonder that expensive highly profitable chemotherapy and infusions are the treatment of choice as there is no financial incentive to learn or to give prudent advice on proper nutrition of the patient. The magic bullet approach is very profitable, but from all objective views not very effective in most cases. Dr. Peter Ubel MD, the author of *Critical Decisions* and *Free Market Madness* said – *"Giving physicians an incentive to prescribe expensive drugs is bad medicine!"* The rationale for "buy and bill" is that it provides convenience to patients, better monitoring of side effects, and improves doctor patient relationships. (9)

LIMITING EXPOSURE TO HARMFUL CHEMICALS

A good way to reduce your chemical exposure is by investigating your home cleaning products. Do not be fooled by the "organic" labeling on some cleaning products. Household cleaning products are not regulated by the Organic Foods Production Act. Labels such as "Natural", "Eco-friendly", and "Non-toxic" are not to be trusted.

Just like food products, you should read the labels of cleaning products. If the product does not have a complete list on the packaging, simply avoid purchasing it. There are certainly some catch-words that should raise a red flag. "Poison" is a real strong word and anything containing this label should not be in your home. "Danger" is another word that should clue the buyer in on product toxicity. Danger and poison labels usually indicate the most toxic types of household cleaners. Familiarity with cleaning products somehow has made us think that they are safe. Just because they are easily purchased does not make them safe.

"Warning" labels are moderately toxic in comparison to danger and or poison labels. Products bearing a "caution" label are less toxic than products containing the warning label. Some of the most toxic chemicals used for household cleaning are toilet bowl cleaners, bleach, oven cleaners, and ammonia products.

Combinations of cleaners that contain chlorine and ammonia can produce very toxic fumes like chlorine gas, a gas that was used in WWII. You must remember that cleaning products are chemicals. It's much safer to buy plant based cleaners as opposed to petroleum based cleaners. The plant based cleaners may cost a little more but they are a much better choice when it comes to reducing your total chemical exposure. If you are chronically sick or tired, removing chemicals from your house may prove to be a vital step in recovering your health.

Laundry detergents contain phosphates and surfactants. These chemicals end up in the sewer systems and ultimately back into the environment. They don't break down during the processing at most municipal water purification plants. Given adequate concentrations, these chemicals are deadly to marine life. Phosphates encourage the overgrowth of algae in streams which can be deadly for fish and other animal life.[10]

These chemicals are also found in dishwashing liquids. Laundry and dishwashing detergents that are free of phosphate and surfactants are easy to find. I have documented some places that totally biodegradable phosphate and surfactant free products can be found on regenesis4health.com.

Oven cleaners and drain cleaners are other sources of toxic chemicals in the home. They contain sodium hydroxide and lye. The aerosol types of oven cleaners when inhaled and are very corrosive to delicate respiratory tissues. When it comes to cleaning ovens, natural mixtures of baking soda, soap, and distilled vinegar combined with a little water will do the trick. You will need to supply the elbow grease.

Air fresheners are very common chemicals found in most homes, the most common forms are the aerosols used to reduce odors in the house. These chemicals are notorious for contributing to, or causing headaches, rashes, dizziness, asthma, coughing, and other symptoms. Children are particularly vulnerable to these chemicals.[11]

Paints, carpets, mattresses, furniture, and certain fabrics also "out-gas" chemicals over time. Formaldehyde is a common chemical used in building products, furniture, and clothing products.

Paints are known to out-gas formaldehyde and benzene long after they have dried. These chemicals have been linked to certain types of cancers, asthma, and other health problems.[12] Paints that are free of volatile organic compounds (VOC's) can be purchased at most major paint supply houses. These products are a little more expensive, but are worth it when it comes to reducing total chemical exposure in the home. Benjamin Moore is one of my favorite paint companies with one of the largest selection of colors available in reduced, or VOC free paints. Their website is: *store.benjaminmoore.com*. Sherwin-Williams manufacturers several different lines in VOC free paints as well. Make the extra investment and know that you are investing in your long term health and also the health of your family.

Cotton or wool clothing is less likely to contain formaldehyde that is found in wrinkle free clothing and bedding products. This popular type of cloth, containing resins that produce the wrinkle free effect, can cause contact dermatitis in sensitive individuals. Out-gassing of formaldehyde occurs with draperies, furniture fabrics, carpeting, and a host of wood products like paneling. If you have ever walked into a new mobile home, travel trailer, or some RV's, and experienced burning eyes, this is most likely due to out-gassing of formaldehyde.

...the average woman will use twelve products with over 168 chemicals in them just getting ready for work.

When it comes to body care, the average woman will use twelve products with over 168 chemicals in them getting ready for work! Men will use six products with 85 chemicals in them. These facts are from the Environmental Working Group.[13] The chemicals in these products can work together to produce an accumulated effect often called "the toxic burden". There are many offenders. Let's take a look at a few of the most common ones.

Sodium Lauryl Sulfate (SLS) or Sodium Laureth Sulfate is in a lot of soaps, shampoos, and toothpaste. SLS is a foaming agent and a surfactant which behaves similarly to soap. A by-product of the production of these surfactants is 1-4 dioxane[14] recognized by the International Agency for Research on Cancer (IARC) as a group 2B suspect carcinogen.[15] I don't know about you, but I don't want to put anything in my hair, on my body, or in my mouth that is "suspect in causing cancer". I would much rather use products that are not "suspect".

Parabens are chemical preservatives used in common everyday body care products like toothpaste, deodorants, shampoo, soap, body lotions, and some food products. Bacterial infections from spoiled body care products in the 50's prompted the use of preservatives in these products.(16) Parabens are cheap and effective. They go by names such as propylparaben, butylparaben, and methylparaben. A study done in 2004 at the University of Reading in the UK suggested a possible link between parabens and breast cancers.(17) As usual, more studies are suggested. I have a suggestion: Use paraben-free cosmetics and beauty care products. The words "possible" and "suspect", are not words that I want to wait for the FDA to clarify for me, especially since there are wonderful paraben free products available.

I want to bring up Bisphenol-A (BPA) again as it is a particularly pervasive chemical. It is used in baby bottles and other plastics. It has been known for some time that BPA is an endocrine disruptor. It has been linked to prostate cancer, and possibly breast cancer, as well as sexual abnormalities. Over 700 studies involving the toxic effect of BPA have been done. A study published in *Reproductive Toxicology*, found that infants and fetuses were the most vulnerable to adverse effects from BPA and other chemicals.(18) Don't let your children drink out of plastic containers!! You shouldn't use them either.

BPA was declared a toxic chemical by the Canadian government's Health Canada in 2008. I thought I would go to the FDA's website myself and see what their opinion on BPA is:

The FDA article "Overview" says:

BPA (Bisphenol-A) is a chemical used in certain food contact materials and first approved by FDA in the early 1960's. In recent years, concerns have been raised about BPA's safety. In August 2008, FDA released a draft report finding that BPA remains safe in food contact materials.

On October 31, 2008, a subcommittee of FDA's science board raised questions about whether FDA's review had adequately considered the most recent scientific information available. On Jan 15, 2010 and again on March 30, 2012, the FDA issued an *interim update on BPA*. For recommendations for the public, see *Bisphenol A (BPA) Information for Parent* on the Department of Health and Human Services Web site.

On the same page as the overview is a section called "Response to Petition of BPA".

On October 28, 2008, The National Resources Defense Council (NRDC) submitted a citizen petition regarding BPA. The petition requested that the Commissioner of Food and Drugs:

*Issue a regulation prohibiting the use of BPA in human food and packaging, and

*Revoke all regulations permitting the use of any food additive that may result in BPA becoming a component of food.

On March 30, 2012, the FDA denied this request in accordance with 21 CRG 10.30 (e). In its response, the FDA stated that:

*The information provided in the citizen petition was not sufficient to persuade FDA to initiate this rulemaking.

*The most appropriate course of action at this time is to continue scientific study and review all of the new evidence regarding the safety of BPA.

*Although FDA was not persuaded by the date and information in the NRDC citizen petition to initiate rulemaking to revoke the food additive approvals for BPA, FDA will continue in its broader and

more comprehensive review of emerging data and information on BPA. Depending on the results, any of these studies or data could influence FDA's assessment and future regulatory decisions about BPA.

Source (http;/www.fda.gov/FoodiIngredientsPackaging/ucm166145.htm). (19)

I am a little uneasy about the FDA taking this kind of stance on BPA given the massive amount of credible information that is available. I don't knowingly use anything containing BPA. I certainly would not want a pregnant woman or child to be exposed to it either. Just a side note, BPA is found on most cash register and credit card receipts! I want to make the point again, if you work in a place that requires handling receipts, you should wear thin protective gloves if possible.

It requires effort, thought, money, and some research to rid your home and therefore your body of toxic chemicals. When it comes to your health, it's worth it in the long run. A lot of chronic health problems are caused by long term chemical exposure. One of the early books written on this subject is *Detoxify or Die*, by Dr. Sherry Rodgers.(20) Another good book, and there are many, on toxicity in household products is *What's in This Stuff?* by Patricia Thomas.(21)

Exposure to toxins begins before birth as many of the toxins contained in a mother's body care products, food chemicals, medicines, even the air she breathes crosses the placenta into the developing fetus. (22)

Talcum powder has a significant link to ovarian cancer; according to Dr. Epstein we have known this fact for many years.(23) I do not recall ever seeing a warning of this fact on any talcum powder containers. I can remember the smell of baby shampoo, and I certainly remember the talcum powder cloud my mother created when caring for my younger siblings, just as she had done with me. Where is the FDA on this? Do not count on the FDA to protect you! The FDA basically allows the cosmetic and body care industry to police itself. Talk about putting the fox in charge of the hen-house. Self-regulation basically means no regulation at all.

From his book *Toxic Beauty*, Dr. Epstein writes:

> Manufacturers are not required to provide proof of the safety of any personal-care or cosmetic ingredient, let alone its effectiveness, to the government or anyone else. Safety is the responsibility of manufacturers; the FDA allows them to use their own judgment about whether a product is safe or not, in effect putting them on the "honor system".
>
> As should be clear from the evidence presented in this book (Toxic Beauty), the FDA's presumption that industry will exercise responsibility is naïve at best and negligent at worst. (24)

Also according to Dr. Epstein at the time he wrote his *Toxic Beauty*, the body care industry had only discontinued three ingredients of known toxins from body care products. There are over 10,000 chemicals used in body care products and they have eliminated only three! (25) How safe do you feel now? Pay attention to what I am telling you here. This stuff is real and it has a cumulative effect on your health and the health of your family. I would suggest you investigate your soaps, shampoos, baby care products, make-up, lipstick, nail polish, mascara, body lotions, hairspray, and everything you come in contact with. Beauty parlors and nail salons can be very toxic places.

Start cleaning up the landfill of toxins that exists in your living space.

Start cleaning up the landfill of toxins that exists in your living space. You know rats don't cause landfills, however rats will show up if you build a landfill. The rats I am talking about are the scary diseases that end up on our doorsteps like cancer, MS, Parkinson's and others.

If you still don't believe our agencies are failing us, and you really want to learn more about the regulatory failure regarding body care products, Dr. Epstein wrote another great book *The Safe Shoppers Bible.*[26] I would suggest you pick up a copy and read it for yourself. This is the third book written by Dr. Epstein that I have recommended in this chapter, obviously he is a tireless crusader and his books are real eye openers.

We have come to the false belief that our government agencies are protecting us. We believe and trust they are giving us proper warnings about the many products we use on a daily basis. I'm going to say it again. "It is up to you to take care of your health and the health of your children". <u>Do not</u> count on governmental agencies to do this for you.

Don't put anything on your skin that you would be afraid to eat! Be aware of what you put on your body, what you wash your hair with, and the types of makeup and hair care products you use. Be aware of the chemicals you use to clean your house. Don't put your bare hands in kerosene or gasoline. DO NOT SPRAY WD 40 ON YOUR JOINTS!!! Know that the things you buy like drapes, carpets, paint, and furniture can have long term health consequences. Clean up the environment that you spend most of your life in and you, and your family, will be much healthier as a result.

SUMMARY

Here is the plan so far. Drink pure water, eat wheat free, and gluten free foods, eliminate simple sugars, use quality oils and fats. Improve your cooking methods. I hope you look at your potential chemical exposure in your cleaning and household products and your foods. Hopefully your shopping routes are starting to change to accommodate purchasing better quality household products, body care products and foods for you and your family.

8

Warning Lights

"The Doctor of the future will give no medicine but pay particular attention to the care and maintenance of the human frame."
Thomas Edison

THOMAS EDISON'S QUOTE appears in a lot of health books. How about this phrase-"Whatever a man soweth, that shall he also reap." These phrases are timeless and apply to the theme of this book. Most of the health problems that people have, they created. I want you to live free from the need for drugs; I want you to understand where health comes from, not just where disease comes from. I have been a practicing Doctor of Chiropractic (DC) since Dec. of 1997. It seems that a lot of my fellow practitioners who write books omit that they are chiropractors. They just call themselves doctor this or doctor that. I am very proud of being a chiropractor. It is a very misunderstood profession, and one of the best kept secrets in health care.

Chiropractic is the largest drug-free health care delivery system in the world. It's totally American made. It began in Davenport, Iowa in 1895 created by the first chiropractor, D. D. Palmer. He was certainly not the first person to pay particular attention to the human frame. Hippocrates spoke extensively about the human frame and performed "bone-setting".

Over the years, chiropractic has gone through a lot of changes, as have all of the health care disciplines. Chiropractic health care is constantly evolving and improving. The central premise of chiropractic has never changed, that is "the power (or intelligence) that created the body, heals the body".

In spite of a deliberate attempt by the American Medical Association (AMA) and several other organizations to destroy chiropractic over the years [1], there are approximately 70,000 Doctors of Chiropractic in the US.

Chiropractors can be found in almost every country in the world. While the relationship of chiropractors and allopathic (MD's) doctors is improving, there is still much work to do on both sides. Patients would ultimately benefit if only the bridges of understanding could be built between all health care disciplines. I know a lot of hard working, caring MD's, nurses, and all kinds of therapists. I refer my patients to them if they need specific types of interventions. I just wish all the crazy politics would go away, but this is America and we love our politics.

Most chiropractors approach health from a vitalistic point of view. We feel that a person is more than the sum of his or her parts. There is a vital energy that exists in all of us. This energy, that most chiropractors call innate intelligence, is what maintains us throughout our lifetime. Some people call it God, some call it vital energy, and there are other terms used for it. I don't care what you call it as long as you understand that it exists. I would like to follow this with two quotes. The first is a quote from Stephenson Chiropractic textbook, the second one by Max Planck, the originator of quantum theory, and a Nobel Prize winner in physics.

"A universal intelligence is in all matter and it gives to it all its properties and actions thus maintaining it in existence." Robert Stephenson [3]

"As a man who has devoted his whole life to the most clear headed science, to the study of matter, I can tell you as a result of my research about atoms this much: There is no matter as such! All matter originates by virtue of a force. We must assume behind this force the existence of a conscious and intelligent mind. This mind is the matrix of all matter." Max Planck (4)

If you cut yourself, your inborn intelligence heals the cut. It tells you how many times to breathe, it makes red blood cells, manufactures enzymes, insulin, adrenaline, neurotransmitters, and it performs thousands of other vital body functions. It gives you pain if there is a problem and sends out all kinds of warning signals that a lot of us just ignore. This intelligence that Planck and Stephenson spoke of must flow freely across the nerves of our bodies if we are to enjoy true health. This is what chiropractors do; keep the nerve energy free from interference by correcting spinal misalignments. Chiropractic is not all about back pain, it is much more than that. Find a good chiropractor to keep your spine in proper alignment, this will allow your body's innate intelligence to flow across your nerve system without interference. A chiropractic treatment is called a "spinal adjustment". A famous quote from Hippocrates is – "Look well to the spine for the cause of disease".

Several years ago, I was driving on the interstate about 75 miles from my home. I was on the way to one of my favorite vacation destinations when the "service engine" light came on. Here I am, 75 miles from home, going somewhere for rest and relaxation, and this dilemma begins.

What should I do? Should I keep on driving and have it checked at my vacation destination? Should I turn around, go back home, and switch vehicles, and consume half a day? Should I pull over at the first available place to have a mechanic, that I do not know or trust, check it for me?

Whatever the case, there was a significant amount of worry over a simple light on my dashboard. When a warning light in your car comes on, you get concerned and immediately start thinking of the prudent thing to do. You take the necessary action as soon as possible. For some reason it is not the same when the "warning lights" come on for your own body. Your body is the vehicle that you must live in for your entire life. You can't trade it in!

It seems to me that a lot of people take better care of their cars than they do their bodies. We largely ignore our own warning lights. Some folks don't even know that they are being given a warning by their bodies. When we do get some warnings, like pain, we just cover it up with medicines and go on. Chronic pain is a warning light! Chronic sickness is a warning light! Obesity, stiffness, skin rashes, and hypertension are all examples of warning lights!

> My patients will tell you that I draw crazy pictures all of the time to help them understand things. I obviously couldn't find icons for human symptoms on a car dashboard so I just drew them myself. When my patients read this book I know they will chuckle when they see my drawings, you may chuckle too, it's okay.

Going to the doctor and getting a drug to reduce the warning light or make the light go out is not fixing the problem. It's like putting a piece of tape over the light and thinking that everything is fine. If you have high blood pressure and take medication, your blood pressure comes down. If it solved the problem, after a while you could stop taking the medicine and your blood pressure would be normal, but this is not the case. Medicines don't always solve the problem; many times they drive the problems deeper. A lot of medicines create new problems adding to the old ones that have not been fixed. The cycle gets bigger as the warning lights of your body continue to be taped over. The original conditions are suppressed and driven further into the body, and the symptom patterns change. True healing occurs from the top down (from the brain down to the body) and from the inside out; suppressing symptoms goes against your body's natural healing instincts. This is a holistic healing concept called "Hering's Law of Cure". (5)

When it comes to being unhealthy, a good question to keep asking is "Why". Why do I have hypertension? Why do my joints ache? Why am I gaining so much weight? Why do I have psoriasis or eczema? I see a lot of patients who never ask "Why". I know this because they take medicines for things that I know can be fixed without drugs and yet these patients will take these drugs for the rest of their lives. The current medical system we have in America never seems to ask "Why" enough. Modern medicines cover up a lot of warning lights.

Modern medicines cover up a lot of warning lights.

America's medical system is arguably the best in the world when it comes to trauma or emergency intervention. However, when it comes to chronic degenerative diseases, their only approach seems to be medicines, various therapies or surgeries but little to no emphasis on the true nutritional needs of the human body. While they understand trauma injuries and disease, their methods of promoting health through medicines, I feel, are flawed. Medicines do not create health; people who take a lot of medicines are not "healthy".

Being and staying healthy requires effort and understanding, which starts by identifying what you have, then asking why or how you developed that particular problem or disease. In order to regain your health, you must eliminate the things that you are doing or being exposed to. Learn how to turn your warning lights off by finding and fixing the source of the problem.

Learn how to turn your warning lights off by finding and fixing the source of the problem.

Chiropractic is a total body health and wellness healing art. The ultimate goal of chiropractic care is for your inborn innate intelligence to flow freely across your nerve system without interference, for your entire life. Most of the patients I see have come to me because they are experiencing some kind of pain. I understand this and use the opportunity to educate them that pain is a warning light. There may be underlying health problems that are causing their pain. Other than an obvious recent trauma, I can usually connect past traumas, lifestyle and dietary habits to their problem. Once I make that connection for the patient, they begin to understand that it's their lifestyle, or their poor choices, that are contributing to their health challenges.

Joint Pain

In a lot of my cases, there is a skeletal or spinal column component that can be corrected using chiropractic treatments to gently realign the joints of the spine or extremities. If these realignments do not hold, that signals to me that there may be underlying issues that need to be addressed. These underlying causes can be nutritional, stress related, or emotionally triggered. It has been my experience that a lot of joint and back pain is caused by chronic dehydration. Simply removing man made beverages, consuming pure water, and adding proper supplementation may help to fix the problem.

The main focus of a chiropractor is the relationship of the human spine to overall health. The spine contains the spinal cord that is an extension of the brain. The brain and spinal cord are called the "Central Nervous System". The nerves that exit the spine create the "Peripheral Nervous System". The nerves that exit the skull (cranial nerves) and the spine go to virtually every part of the body. If there is interference with the nerve transmission either to or from the brain, your body cannot function at 100%. Making corrections to the spine can eliminate interference with vital nerve transmission. This in turn can certainly correct muscle weakness, pain, and organ dysfunction.

The same nerves that go to your muscle and skeletal systems also supply your organs with this vital nerve energy. That is the part of the chiropractic story most people never hear. You may have a back ache but depending on where the problem is with your spine, it could be the same nerve that also supplies your heart, colon, kidneys or some other organ with vital nerve energy. Chiropractic adjustments help to keep vital nerve energy flowing at optimal levels. This is why it is so important to take care of your spine. A good chiropractor can help you maintain optimal spinal and neurological function for a lifetime. It is not all about back pain!

If there is interference with the nerve transmission either from the brain or to the brain, your body cannot function at 100%.

Taking care of your body including your frame, is a major part of living a healthy life. Your body is the vehicle you have been given to take you through your entire life. Of course, being a chiropractor, I recommend that you have regular chiropractic checkups and treatments in order to maintain your structural body. Structure and function are intimately linked.

Massage therapy, yoga, stretching, meditation, and relaxation techniques are other worthwhile things to learn how to utilize. Spend a little time and money on yourself from time to time. When someone asks what you want for your birthday or anniversary, tell them you would like a professional massage. This is a great gift.

Taking care of your skeletal system is as important as having your blood checked annually or maintaining your teeth every six months. If your car goes out of alignment, your tires and bushings can wear out. Likewise, if your spine or other joints are out of alignment, your discs (bushings) and/or joints can wear down as well. You can't go to NAPA or Auto Zone and get some new bushings for your spine! Joint replacement surgeries are becoming common in the lexicon of most Americans. Joints have to be replaced mainly due to people being overweight, malnourished, dehydrated, and mineral deficient, especially the minerals calcium, silica, and sulfur.

More specifically, let's point out some of your body's warning lights and signals. One of my favorite examples is temperature. If the temperature light on your automobile dashboard comes on, the water temperature is too high. If not attended to, this can damage your engine. When your temperature goes up, it usually means that there is an infection of some kind in your body. Elevating temperature is a healthy response and is the way your body deals with infection. In most cases, the more severe the infection, the higher the temperature will go. This is the innate wisdom of your body at work, it knows what to do. But most Americans don't heed the warnings because they can't afford to miss work, so they grab the aspirin to lower their temperature and go to work anyway. They ignore the warning light and chemically alter the natural response of their inborn intelligence. Being a recovering work-a-holic myself, I completely understand why we do this.

WATER TEMP

We fix our cars, but we will not allow our body's internal healing mechanisms to work as intended. Certainly, very high fevers should be properly attended to by a health care practitioner. Most of the time, medicines are taken for normally elevated body temperatures. It would be wiser to let the fever run its course and respect the needs of the body for rest and hydration.

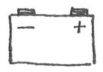

Low Battery

What happens if the battery or alternator warning light comes on in the car? If it is not attended to, you will not be able to start your car and may possibly get stranded. A fully charged battery and a properly functioning charging system is crucial for your car. What happens if your battery runs down? What if you are not adequately "charged" every day? Fatigue or a general lack of energy and motivation are warning signals. How do Americans respond to these warnings? They consume Monster, Amp energy drinks, Mountain Dew, Coke, or some other caffeinated beverage like coffee or cappuccinos. How about the popular 5 hour energy drinks? This comes from the false idea that health or energy comes from a bottle. A properly nourished and healthy body has adequate energy without stimulants.

Fatigue is one of the most common complaints I hear as a health care practitioner. Decreased energy, lack of motivation, and brain fog are all signs that could be linked to a chronic health problem. Adrenal exhaustion, cortisol problems, dehydration, vitamin and/or mineral deficiencies, food allergies, poor diet, excessive stress, thyroid problems, and many other things can cause these types of symptoms. Americans ignore the warning signals

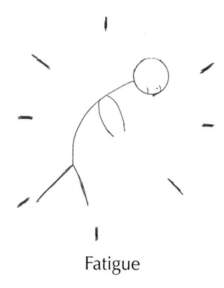

Fatigue

and just write them off as a caffeine deficiency, old age, or what-ever. Once again we have placed a piece of tape over our body's warning light.

It should go without saying, but I am going to say it anyway: Avoid the landmines in life. Don't smoke, don't walk out in front of oncoming traffic, don't drink and drive. I know people that work constantly on their health and then text while they drive. This makes no sense.

Smoking is one of the unhealthiest things you can do. It is a major risk factor in almost every known condition or disease associated with aging. There are many risky behaviors such as doing meth-amphetamines, cocaine, heroin, or jumping off a cliff. Cigarettes are readily available which makes smoking easy to do. Not too long ago, in the late 30's, 40's, and 50's, magazine ads used pictures of doctors to assure consumers that cigarettes were safe. They would make claims that doctors smoked their brands more often than any other cigarettes. These ads also appeared in the Journal of The American Medical Association (JAMA) and other medical journals. The Medical profession has had a long relationship with the tobacco industry in America.

Smoking places incredible stress on all body systems. Cigarettes are fair targets for excise taxes because they place a very heavy burden on the cost of health care. Cigarettes can cost $10.00 a pack and yet people still use them! How much does this impact their monthly budget, and more importantly, how is affecting their health? Every cigarette robs you of your health and drives another nail into your coffin.

Cigarettes contain seven thousand chemicals, some of which are known carcinogens.(9) The warnings on cigarette packs are largely ignored in the same way people ignore their health warning lights. Because tobacco has been one of the staple crops of this country since its founding, it is unlikely that the tobacco problem is going to go away any time soon.

Obesity is another warning. One of the most obvious warnings that you are unhealthy is being overweight. Being morbidly obese is a flashing red warning light. It is easy to predict things that happen to obese patients: disc problems, knee and hip replacements, strokes, heart attacks, cancer,

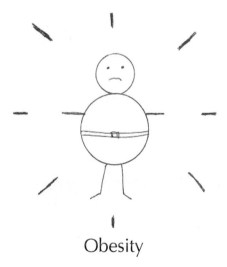

Obesity

and diabetes. I go over these potential problems all the time hoping to motivate my overweight patients to start their journey towards good health. It's a long journey, but worth the effort. Those are my values which unfortunately not everyone shares. The reasons that have caused a patient to become obese must be overcome before any lasting progress can be made. For a lot of people, the reasons they are obese are emotional, and these can be the most difficult to overcome.

There is a restaurant in my home town that features home cooking. I frequently go there for breakfast and get farm fresh eggs cooked in butter. A collection of guys like me eat there on a regular basis. We sit at the large table next to a big picture window. I call us the "Breakfast Club". We have a heavy equipment operator, a heavy equipment mechanic, a contractor, a professor type, a tree specialist, a preacher, a couple of retirees, some occasional visitors, and me the chiropractor. This makes for some very interesting conversation.

One morning I was sitting there and one of the regulars asked me how my book was coming along. One of the retired guys (that I do not know very well) chimed in and told me that it didn't matter what he ate, or what kind of diet he tried, because of his genetics. He was right, but for the wrong reason. The food choices he makes influences his genetic survival instincts. If you consume empty calories, you do not adequately nourish your body. Your genes perceive this as starvation, a very strong survival "instinct".[10] The instinctive genetic response then calls for more food so his hunger is never really satisfied as long as he continues to make the wrong food choices. Conversely, if he consumes high nutrient dense foods, his genes are satisfied that this basic survival need is being met and the call to eat is normal. The point here is that poor quality foods make you crave more food. This creates a never ending hunger merry-go-round orchestrated by your genetic survival mechanisms.

...poor quality foods make you crave more food.

He ordered two gravy biscuits with fried potatoes and pancakes; then he smothered his pancakes with margarine and high fructose corn syrup. Just before that, he put five packs of sugar and some hydrogenated powdered creamer in his coffee. I could not for the life of me make him understand that it's his food choices that were making him obese. He could shut off the relentless genetic call to eat in a few days with the proper food choices. We went back and forth making our cases like two armchair lawyers. I eventually left him alone because it didn't matter what I said to him. His addiction to sugar and refined carbs along with his emotional need to eat this way, are stronger than his desire to be healthy. He is on a self-propelled genetic merry-go-round that he does not know how to stop. I hope that I planted a seed in that conversation that may take root in the future.

Your genetic code is what gives you dark or light hair and blue or brown eyes. It makes you tall or short, big or small boned, male or female, but it does not make you obese. The nutritional signals that you send to your genes by your food choices <u>will</u> make you obese. I see entire families that are all obese. What I know about them is they all have the same eating habits. This is a familial trait, not a genetic trait. Children who grow up eating poor quality foods, because of the family lifestyle, socioeconomic status, or both, will tend to continue that lifestyle into adulthood. There is a very strong chance that they will pass their lifestyle along to their children as well. Call it what you want, but in the end it is not caused by faulty genetics, it's lifestyle.

The point I have been trying to make through this entire chapter, is that your body only has a few ways to "talk" to you, to let you know when something is wrong. It's normal to have a fever if you are sick or diarrhea if you have an intestinal flu. It's normal to bruise or clot if you hit something. Vomiting is a perfectly healthy response; your body is trying to expel a toxin of some kind. The chronic long term symptoms (warning lights) are what I want to make you aware of. If you ignore long term problems, you are most likely going to experience at least a gradual decline in your health, and at worst, a tragic or life altering event. Do not ignore or cover up your warning lights.

9 Supplementation

*"Leave your drugs in the chemist's pot if
you can heal the patient with food,"*
Hippocrates

BY FAR THE largest and most complicated endeavor I have attempted is the journey into the nutritional needs of the human body. It is replete with disagreement, controversy, misinformation, politics, and downright fraud. Opinions and so called "facts" change like the seasons. Environmental, technological, and lifestyle factors are rapidly changing in our culture. This adds a countless variety of constantly evolving factors that must be considered when dealing with patients. Our ever increasing need to mass produce foods because of an expanding world population has created many problems. We are playing with Mother Nature by increasing yields through biotechnologies like genetic engineering and hybridization. There once was an old Chiffon margarine commercial that said "It's not nice to fool Mother Nature". It was meant to be funny and the commercial was very clever, but hydrogenated foods like margarine have contributed immensely to the poor health of our nation.

"It's not nice to fool Mother Nature."

The soils used in commercial mass production of foods are so exhausted that there is virtually no way to get the required amount of minerals from them needed to achieve and maintain good health.[1] Our proteins from commercial meat sources are now laced with growth hormones and chemicals.[2] Animals have been force-fed foods that they don't normally eat. Cows, for example, will eat corn but it's not their preferred food. They like naturally grazing in healthy green pastures. The force feeding of corn to cattle in concentrated animal feeding operations (CAFO) has caused a massive shift in omega 6 oils in our beef. Natural, free-range, hormone, and antibiotic free beef, is loaded with omega 3 oils, vitamins and minerals.[3] The point here is that our food supply is so manipulated and devoid of nutrition that it is absolutely necessary to properly supplement it if you want to be healthy.

The top six diseases that kill Americans: [heart disease, cancer, chronic obstructive pulmonary disease, stroke, Alzheimer's and diabetes] have major dietary and lifestyle connections. Most medical doctors do not get anywhere close to the nutritional education they need to properly counsel patients. Dietitians hand out the same diet that doctors have been taught, the prudent diet. This diet has been discredited by so much research it is amazing to me that it is still in use. As of the time this book was written, the old food pyramid is still used on the back of bread packaging. If you were a bread manufacturer or a cereal manufacturer, you would certainly continue to promote the grain based (up to eleven servings of grains a day) prudent diet that is represented by the old food pyramid.

Doctors will refer patients, particularly diabetics, to "programs" designed to instruct them on how to eat healthy. One of my diabetic patients brought me the class handouts from one of these programs. The information was unbelievable and she did not notice any improvement in her diabetes. Her insurance company paid $2,400.00 for one of the classes I mentioned previously. So, if our food supply is terribly lacking in nutrients and our health care providers and dietitians are under educated and ignorant of true nutrition of the human body, how could you ever hope to be really healthy in the current "health care" system no matter how much it costs?

It's almost impossible to determine the truth about health because the facts get lost in dietary dogma and opinions. We see ridiculous commercials on TV, read ads and articles in so-called "health" magazines, and hear conflicting remarks by so-called "experts" on the news.

I was driving down the road one day, the radio news was on and a sound bite came over the air waves. I could not believe what I was hearing. The news anchor said, "An Australian researcher says we may be drinking too much water." I located the quote-

> *Our bodies need about two liters of fluids per day, not two liters of water specifically. In an Editorial in the June issue of Australian and New Zealand Journal of Public Health, Spero Tsindos from La Trobe University, examined why we consume so much water.*
>
> *Mr. Tsindos believes that encouraging people to drink more water is driven by vested in- trests, rather than a need for better health. "Thirty years ago you didn't see a plastic water bottle anywhere, now they appear as fashion accessories... As tokens of instant gratification and symbolism, the very bottle itself is seen as cool and hip. ... We should be telling people that beverages like tea and coffee contribute to a person's fluid needs and despite their caffeine content, do not lead to dehydration."* (4)

Patients will come to me and say "I heard on the radio that coffee and tea will not hurt you. I heard they really do help hydrate you, but you told me to cut out man made beverages." This type of thing has happened to me countless times. Mr. Tsindos is basically asserting that water bottles are fashionable and that the bottled water industry wants you to drink more water so they can increase their profits. Of course they do! So does Pepsi, Coca-Cola, Dr Pepper, Folgers, Ford, Starbucks, McDonalds, Sears, Old Navy, and all corporations that make money by the choices consumers make.

After reading the report in its entirety, I agree with most of the assertions Mr. Tsindos makes. The article went into some history and detail about water consumption theories handed down over the years. But this is not what is heard in the ten second sound bite on the radio.

I am no fan of bottled water as I discussed in Chapter 2, however, Mr. Tsindos assertion that coffee and tea are just as hydrating as pure water is not entirely true. Caffeine in coffee has a significant dehydrating effect. This is just one example of hundreds of crazy things that people hear or see in the media in the form of 10 second sound-bites. One of the most incredible things I see is the rapid, and often dramatic, improvements in health when a patient actually stops drinking man-made beverages, and replaces them with pure water. To move a person from poor health to good health requires proper hydration, this means giving up most of what Americans drink at least in the early phase of the transition.

This little story was meant to demonstrate how we are bombarded with sound bites from so called "experts". These out of context comments often encourage us to make poor dietary choices. Every day I see people who have lived by this kind of advice for thirty or forty years. They come to my office in terrible health.

..we are bombarded with sound bites from so called "experts".

A lot of doctors will say that you get all of your nutritional needs from your diet. These are the same doctors that took a one hour elective class on nutrition in school and belong to the flat earth society. As far back as 1914, the animal industry figured out that vitamins and minerals incorporated into livestock feeds would increase profitability by increasing survival, fertility, and yield (like meat, eggs, and offspring). Along with that, adequate vitamin and mineral supplementation helped to prevent, and in some cases, reverse diseases in livestock and farm animals. In fact, this practice was so successful that almost 900 diseases that affect animals have been eliminated.[5] We Americans are eating our way into our graves so perhaps Purina should make an alfalfa pellet feed with all the right nutrition just for humans. "People Chow!" We could probably prevent and reverse a lot of the common diseases that we suffer from. Maybe a better idea would be to just improve our eating habits, improve our lifestyle, and supplement adequately.

Have you seen what some doctors eat? Chances are good that you eat this way too. Most people do. It's called the Standard American Diet (SAD). I would rather supplement my diet with a full complement of all the nutrients I need. Even if I pee away some of my money, it's better than chronic illness, chemotherapy, bypass surgery, and knee replacements. Many so called "health experts" tell you that vitamins give you expensive urine. I would rather take my chances with expensive urine than have chronic sickness, pay for multiple specialist visits, and/or take prescription drugs for the rest of my life.

These same "experts" will also tell you that you cannot cure disease with vitamins and minerals. How about iron deficiency anemia? That is cured by restoring iron levels (a mineral). Rickets can be caused by vitamin D and calcium deficiencies (vitamins and minerals). Beriberi is a vitamin B-1 deficiency, Scurvy is a vitamin C deficiency, pernicious anemia is a B-12 deficiency, and so on. Calcium deficiency has been linked to 147 conditions. On average there are about 10 diseases that are associated with each of the essential minerals needed by humans. You require 60 minerals for good health.[6] That equals about 600 diseases or conditions associated or linked to mineral deficiencies. Adequate vitamins and minerals are crucial for good health.

Hopefully, when it comes to proper nutrition and adequate supplementation of essential vitamins, minerals, and essential oils, you will not believe your radio, TV advertisers, or under educated doctors and nutritionists. You don't have to believe me either. As with anything in this book, I encourage you to research it for yourself.

I can tell you that when people follow the REGENESIS program including the recommended essential supplementation, they get major improvements in their health. A lot of the health problems that their doctors have been "managing" for years with medications go away.

There is some discussion out there that suggests that supplements are dangerous. A lot of this comes from the FDA, a watch-dog organization (and to some degree, an advocate in my opinion) for the drug companies, not for the vitamin and supplement industry. Do you really think drug companies want you to get well using supplements instead of drugs? From the "Annual Report of the American Association of Poison Control Centers National Poison Data System" (28th annual report), there were no deaths from vitamin and mineral supplements in 2010.(7) On average, 125,000 people die every year from taking FDA approved drugs <u>as prescribed,</u>(8) so there is a real arrogance on the drug industry's part and from doctors in pointing their fingers at supplements. Don't get me wrong, anything can be done to excess including vitamins and you can die from drinking too much water. Quality vitamins taken in a reasonable fashion under direction of an educated health care provider are totally safe. Some vitamins do interact with certain medications and it is up to you to know. Ask your pharmacists and doctors about these concerns if you take prescription medications.

Your body requires around 90 nutrients every day in order to be healthy. This consists of 60 minerals, 16 vitamins, 12 essential amino acids, and 3 essential fatty acids.(9) When it comes to minerals, doctors understand four or five of them. They know about magnesium, calcium, potassium, phosphorous, manganese, and maybe a couple more. They do not understand the importance of trace minerals like germanium, vanadium, gallium, and chromium, there are many others. From the book *Rare Earths Forbidden Cures-*

> There are 75 metals listed in the periodic chart, all of which have been detected in human blood and other body fluids – we know that at least 60 of these metals (minerals) have physiological value for man. Organically not a single function in the human body can take place without at least one mineral or metal co-factor. (10)

Minerals are best absorbed in plant derived form. This means that plants take minerals up from the soil and break them down into very small particles for their use. We consume the plants containing the minerals in their smallest form which makes them highly absorbable. Plant derived and colloidal minerals (in a suspension of water) are highly metabolically active. They are by far the preferred method of supplemental consumption of these very important nutrients.(11) Minerals are important co-factors in thousands of various biological reactions that take place in your body every day. Americans are more deficient in minerals than any other class of nutrients. Proper mineral supplementation in a highly absorbable form, including rare earth minerals, is one of the major keys to regaining your health.

Americans are more deficient in minerals than any other class of nutrients.

In the early 1900's, wood stoves began to be replaced by gas and electric appliances. The ashes from wood stoves were no longer being spread onto the garden soils. Wood ashes are very high in mineral content. This switch to modern, convenient, and cleaner gas and electric appliances has contributed greatly to the mineral deficiencies we see in the population today.

One mineral in particular that is ignored or misunderstood by most doctors, nutritionists, and certainly the general public, is sulfur. Like a lot of minerals found in the soil, sulfur has been depleted over the years by industrial farming practices. In the mid 1950's, nitrogen based synthetic chemical fertilizers began being used in commercial agriculture. This had a devastating effect on the sulfur content of our farm soils. This farming practice caused a major sulfur deficiency in our food supply and consequently, a significant sulfur deficiency in humans.

Sulfur is not stored in your body and must be consumed daily. It is a major component of amino acids which are the building blocks of the body. Patients with arthritis, allergies, cancer, asthma, skin problems and general connective tissue disorders can benefit significantly from pure crystalline sulfur supplementation. [12]

Eggs, nuts, meats, dairy, garlic, and onions, are all rich in sulfur. Doctors have been vilifying eggs for decades, contributing to the deficiency of sulfur in the population.

Sulfur is an oxygenator, meaning that it helps increase oxygen uptake by the cells of the body. Most cancer cells are anaerobic and do not like oxygen. Cancer rates have skyrocketed in the past 50 to 60 years. I wonder if there is a potential connection. Think about it, we have significant mineral deficiencies along with sulfur deficiencies that decrease oxygenation to our cells. We consume excessive amounts of flour products and sugars that increase fermentation rates. Remember from a previous chapter, Otto Warburg postulated that cancer was caused by decreased oxygenation and increased fermentation. This could be an area of research for a potential cancer treatment or cure. One would think so, but most likely this is not going to happen as sulfur and other minerals are natural and there would be no money to be made. Companies wealthy enough to conduct very expensive research cannot apply patent law to natural minerals.

There is significant evidence that taking crystalline MSM sulfur minimizes the effects of chemotherapy and radiation, and even decreases cancer cell counts. MSM sulfur has been shown to benefit patients with Lymphoma. (13)

Sulfa drugs and sulfur are not the same thing. A lot of people are afraid of taking sulfur supplements because they have had a reaction to a sulfa drug. Sulfur is essential to human health and should not be confused with "sulfa" drugs. I have posted a good source of crystalline MSM on regenesis4health.com.

Rare Earths Forbidden Cures, is a great source of information on minerals, where they come from, and the history around their discovery.

The basic functions of life itself cannot be performed without minerals, either as a major part of the function or as a catalytic co-factor (i.e. RNA, DNA, sub-cellular and digestive enzymes and the utilization of vitamins) ...Simply said, minerals are the currency of life. (14)

Given the poor state of our nation's food supply, and the over farming of our lands, it is impossible to get these nutrients every day, particularly minerals, without supplementing them.

Pica is a condition caused by mineral deficiencies. If you own horses and know what "cribbing" is, this is a form of pica. Horses will eat the wooden fences, or anything around them that is wood, for the mineral content it contains. Farmers and horse owners recognize this and have found that simple mineral supplementation with feeds and/or mineral blocks for a few days stops this behavior. (15)

Americans suffer from pica as well. Chewing ice is a form of pica and indicates an iron deficiency. Craving salty foods is also a form of pica. A lot of Americans eat salty foods while they watch TV in the evenings to satisfy their salt cravings. It's pica that makes you look through your refrigerator 20 minutes after you have eaten a meal. How could you possibly be hungry? The answer is that your meal did not contain adequate minerals, and the resulting pica is what has you rummaging around for more to eat. The odds are that if you didn't get enough minerals at meal time, there are no minerals in your refrigerator either. Most, if not all Americans, are deficient in the 60 minerals needed daily for good health.

It's pica that makes you look through your refrigerator 20 minutes after you have eaten a meal.

Extreme cases of pica involve consuming things like paint chips, leather, dirt, paper products, glass, and other very strange things.

Vitamins are best consumed in their natural state, preferably in the form of organically grown foods. Most commercial vitamins are synthetic and are very poorly absorbed. They contain food colorings, wax like substances, and emulsifiers that are often left over by-products of some other food production industry. The last time I checked, food colorings are not essential to human health, neither is carnuba wax.

On the REGENESIS program, it's important not to consume carbonated beverages as this tends to disrupt stomach acid which is very important for the absorption of minerals.(16) This is another reason I do not allow soft drinks of any kind on the program. Caffeine also interferes with the absorption of minerals. Phytates from grains, nuts and beans also interfere with mineral absorption. Soaking or sprouting grains, nuts, and beans significantly decrease the phytate content. The over use of wheat and wheat products in America has created a massive malabsorption problem in the population (because of the phytate content and the inflammation potential). If you continue to use wheat products and foods that contain phytates you will never be able to properly absorb nutrients, even if you supplement them. This is one of the reasons the wheat and phytate issue is so important.

Amino acids are the building blocks of the body. They are used by the body to construct the proteins necessary for life. It makes sense that these vital nutrients are produced by the breakdown of protein rich foods. You must consume adequate essential amino acids daily. Nine of the twenty amino acids used in the body are considered "essential", meaning your body cannot manufacture them. It is hard but not impossible to get all of the amino acids you need on a vegetarian diet. Unfortunately, rice, corn, and beans (the way vegetarians get their amino acids), are not really allowed on the REGENESIS program for reasons previously explained. Lentils are allowed in small single portions and are a very good vegetable source of essential amino acids but are lacking adequate amounts of one of the essential amino acids, methionine [17]. I always recommend supplementation that includes essential amino acids. Then there is no doubt.

Three of the 90 nutrients your body needs are essential fatty acids Omega 3, 6, and 9. Oils that we consume should be the ones found in nature, as close to their natural form as possible. Wild caught salmon, tuna, deep sea fish, free range meats, including beef, chicken and wild game, such as bison, turkey, and deer meats are all rich in these fatty acids in appropriate balance. When red meat is taken from free range animals it is rich in omega 3 fats [18], Americans generally consume a lot more omega 6 fatty acids from meats and processed cooking oils as compared to omega 3 fats. Balancing these fats is very important. For general health, I recommend a minimum of a 4:1 ratio of Omega 6 to Omega 3 fatty acids. Current ratios can be as high as 20 or 30:1. Avoiding man-made oils like soy oil, corn oil and others will decrease your intake of Omega 6 fats, increasing intake of fish like salmon and other deep sea fish will increase your intake of Omega 3 fats. Olive oil and macademia nuts contain oleic acid, an omega 9 fat. The REGENESIS program deliberately decreases intake of omega 6 fats as we do far too much of this fat in relation to Omega 3. A diet high in poor quality Omega 6 oils causes inflammation and reducing inflammation is one of the main goals of the REGENESIS program. A well balanced EPA-DHA supplement along with a diet rich in quality balanced fats is essential to good health.

For years now, veterinarians have cured hundreds of diseases in animals using nutritional pellets or formulas. We put salt and mineral blocks out in the fields for our cows to lick to ensure that they are healthy but we do not have minerals or a salt blocks on the kitchen table for our families. Here in Virginia there is little to no selenium in the soil. Selenium, a powerful antioxidant, is a very important mineral for human health and farm animals too. Selenium has strong anti-cancer properties. (19) Local farmers around here use salt blocks with selenium because they know the importance of this vital mineral for the health of their livestock. Many of my patients, including the farmers that know about selenium, admitted to me that they did not take this mineral for themselves. Selenium is an important mineral especially for cancer patients, people with muscular diseases, eye problems, and general overall health. Excess selenium, like any excess, can cause serious problems as well. It is always about proper balance.

The bigger you are, the more nutrition you need. A 250 lb. person needs more supplementation than a 120 lb. person. This idea that a single vitamin taken one time a day works for everyone, is ridiculous. On the REGENESIS program, a 300 lb. person will have to spend more for supplements than a 150 lb. person. It is my experience that once a person stops buying the junk foods and soft drinks that they normally use, they will have more than enough money to pay for their supplements. The cost of a pack of cigarettes a day is more than enough to buy quality supplements. A couple of visits to a specialist of some kind could cost you enough money to buy a year's worth of good supplements.

I have researched and used many different vitamin product lines over the years. There are many good companies that put a lot of time and energy into delivering a quality product. There are also a lot of poor quality vitamins on store shelves. One of my patients brought me her bottle of Co-enzyme Q-10 and bragged that she had purchased it at a local discount store for three dollars. CoQ-10 is a very important nutrient for heart health and several other vital functions. This particular nutrient is very difficult to extract and keep stable over time. I am sure that she was wasting her money on this three dollar no-name supplement that is so important to the health of her heart. If you are taking a statin drug for high cholesterol (like they want almost 20% of Americans to do), I assure you it is depleting your body of Co-enzyme Q-10.

I recommend that supplements have adequate macro and micro minerals as well as trace minerals. They must contain all essential amino acids and the necessary vitamins to make them complete. In addition, essential fatty acids should also be taken daily. These requirements total 90 nutrients. These 90 nutrients are necessary for good health. If someone has a particular problem like diabetes, it becomes necessary to add some other nutrients in larger amounts. Chromium, vanadium, cinnamon, bitter melon, and others can be of great benefit to a diabetic. These nutrients can increase cellular sensitivity to insulin provided all of the necessary co-factors are present. Most co-factors in biological reactions are minerals. Americans are woefully lacking minerals especially trace minerals.

Arthritic patients benefit greatly from supplements that nourish the collagen matrix like sulfur (in the form of crystalline MSM), zinc, vitamin C, and others. Proper supplementation can make all the difference when it comes to recovering your health.

I have patients that will bring grocery bags full of supplements that they take every day. This is not necessary and is usually ill advised. I ask them why they take this or that and I get some interesting answers: "I saw it in a magazine", "My neighbor takes it", "a clerk at the grocery store said it helps her". I can go on and on. This approach is no different than taking over the counter medications, the drugs are being replaced with vitamins. Grocery bags full of vitamins are not necessary, very expensive, and usually inadequate. Vitamins and minerals can be taken to excess, and anything done to excess is unhealthy. Proper dietary changes, along with adequate and quality supplementation is not hard to do.

It is important to know that as you begin to take on healthy habits and add quality supplements, your health markers will start to change. Monitor your blood pressure and your blood sugars closely if you are a diabetic. Tell your primary care provider that you are doing a "health program" if you take prescription medications. Diabetics in particular need to monitor their blood sugars very closely as the program can cause fairly quick changes in blood sugar levels. I usually recommend that you follow the diet for several weeks before adding supplements (with help from your primary care physician). This makes it easier for your body to transition from being dependent on drugs to doing what comes naturally.

Success on the REGENESIS program requires proper and adequate supplementation. Good quality supplements are not cheap. The bigger a person is, the more the nutrients they require. This is one area where you truly do "get what you pay for". For this reason, I usually recommend to my patients that they get fully on the diet before purchasing the nutrients. I want them to be successful, and if they cannot do the diet, the nutrients are not nearly as effective by themselves. The REGENESIS program has three parts: diet, supplementation, and exercise, or more appropriately what I call movement therapy. It is best to start movement therapy after one has initiated the dietary changes, started the nutrient supplementation, and is cleared by their physician (if indicated) to start a mild to moderate exercise program. All are essential in achieving your goal.

In Review

I assume by now you are starting to get the big idea that is the REGENESIS program. You should be drinking pure water, absolutely wheat free and using quality natural fats. You should have eliminated simple sugars. Your diet should be mainly non starchy vegetables, free range eggs and quality cuts of free range meats. Meat servings should be the size of the palm of your hand. Hopefully you have surveyed and started removing the harsh and harmful chemicals from your home and begun the process of cleaning up your "landfill". The addition of quality supplementation is the next big step. My recommendations for quality supplements can be found on the REGENESIS website.

www.regenesis4health.com.

10 | Movement

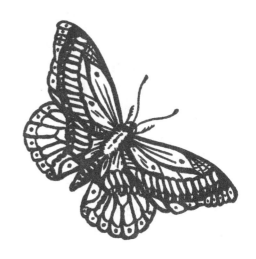

"Movement is a medicine for creating change in a person's physical, chemical, and emotional states."
Carol Welch

WHY IS SO much attention given to exercise? Man is the only animal that exercises. You don't see a lion getting into shape in order to take down a wildebeest for supper. Some people seem to be obsessed with exercise while others could care less. People seem to be all over the spectrum when it comes to exercise. I work on a lot of exercise-o-holics that are in terrible condition. I also see people that don't exercise who are in excellent health. What is a reasonable amount of physical activity or what I just call "movement"?

Man is the only animal that exercises.

Look at some of the primitive societies that still exist in the world, like the Hunza's, Vilacabambans, and Nicoyan's of Costa Rica. They out live us by decades; there are several reasons for that. They do not have convenience stores, nursing homes, public schools, easy access to doctors, chlorinated water, T.V's, phones, fast foods, governmental health agencies like Medicare and the FDA, and they certainly do not have any exercise equipment. You will never see a Hunza tribal member going to Gold's Gym. The Aborigines of Australia do not own Bowflexes, but they actually know how to use a bow and arrow. These long-lived cultures do not experience slow declining health. Most of them live long and very physically active lives and then just die. On the other hand Americans begin to suffer from advancing chronic diseases in their middle ages, leading to declining health. Many Americans have multiple doctors and take multiple medications (polypharmacy) and some of these people languish in nursing facilities for years until they die. These people are factored into longevity studies.

Another thing seen with these long-lived people is that they don't have electricity. They use wood as their primary heat source and they distribute the ashes over their gardens for the mineral content. Do you remember when your grandparents or great grandparents used wood for heat and put the ashes on their gardens? By the way, your great grandparents didn't work out at the gym either.

Long-lived people in primitive societies eat calorie restricted diets from local indigenous foods because that is all they have access to. Many cultures irrigate their crops with mineral rich water from glacier runoff. It hasn't been that long ago that people didn't have gyms where they could go to and work out. Fifty years ago there were very few sports stores, sports drinks, or high protein shakes. What happened? A great book to read on long-lived cultures is *Immortality* by Dr. Joel Wallach and Dr. Ma Lan. [1]

Civilization is advancing and now we enjoy more conveniences than ever. Our lives are becoming easier physically. In turn, this has reduced the meaningful movements that were once necessary for survival; these movements also kept us healthy. Our lives are becoming more difficult in other areas, particularly as far as our health and fitness are concerned.

Not long ago, you couldn't just hop in the car and ride over to your friend's house. You couldn't go pick up a movie or some pizza. If you went somewhere, you had to get on your horse, or hook up the buggy, or just walk. Around the turn of the 20th century there were no skype options, pizza delivery, cell phones, or even pay phones. Today's teenagers do not know what a pay phone is, but they are intimately linked to their personal communication devices. People had gardens and had to work them. There was firewood to cut and stack, and there was hay, corn and other crops that had to be harvested BY HAND! For farming, there were no tractors, baling machines, or hay rakes. People had to move and work just to exist. I am not suggesting that we go back to the horse and buggy days; I just want you to see the contrast.

Early man had to move to survive threats and to rummage around for food. This required various forms of physical exertion like climbing, heavy lifting, and sprinting just to remain alive. The fight or flight response that was required then for survival still exists in our genetic make-up, but is rarely employed now due to our conveniences.

Our lack of movement has made us more unhealthy and overweight. Some of us get the bright idea that we need to do vigorous exercise. We start lifting weights, jogging, and doing other things which most of us are not nourished enough to do. It's here that I differ with a lot of the so called "gurus". I feel it's imperative to have a properly nourished body before beginning any kind of exercise regimen. This takes a few weeks and sometimes longer, depending on the overall health of the individual.

Let's think about this rationally. Whenever you sweat, you are sweating a "soup" mostly made up of minerals and water. Remember from our previous chapter on supplementation, that you need 60 plus minerals every day to be healthy even if you're not working out. Most people don't come anywhere close to meeting nutritional requirements due to a malabsorption syndrome caused by excessive consumption of grains (primarily wheat), foods containing phytates, and a poor overall national food supply that is nutrient deficient. It's asking for trouble to start sweating what little mineral reserve you have by exercising before you are nutritionally ready.

Every year several young high school and college athletes die on the football fields or basketball courts from some "mysterious" heart condition. There is little mystery to this. Our teenagers drink sugar laden sports drinks, soft drinks, energy drinks, coffee, tea, and cappuccinos, but not water. They eat the Standard American Diet and their favorite vegetables are French fries. They rarely supplement their diets adequately with the required minerals, amino acids, essential fatty acids, and vitamins. Every year after hard workouts or strenuous games in sweltering heat, invariably several of these young athletes die from undernourished heart muscle problems (cardiomyopathy). Over time, deficiencies of selenium, vitamin E, essential fatty acids, and other nutrients, combined with excessive stress on an undernourished heart can cause pathological conditions of the heart muscle.

In 2011, a star high school basketball player had just made the shot that won his team the state championship. A few moments later he collapsed and died. When these awful events happen, doctors always wrangle over the possible causes. It almost always seems to be some kind of heart related issue. No kidding? Most young athletes practice and sweat for years and never get the adequate nutrition they need, nor do they replace the minerals they lose. They develop these silent cardiomyopathy heart issues, and a seemingly healthy young athlete suddenly dies.

This cardiomyopathy heart issue is also found in adults. Most adults eat the American way (SAD diet) and are deficient in vitamins and minerals. This is why I never require vigorous exercise on the REGENESIS program. I prefer a slow gradual increase in movement (I particularly like walking initially) in conjunction with proper dietary changes and adequate supplementation.

Extreme conditioning is not rewarded with longevity. When one sweats out essential nutrients for years and never adequately replaces them, cardiomyopathy heart issues can and do occur. Add strenuous workout programs, or jobs working out in the heat for years, and you have a recipe for a cardiomyopathy surprise, a fatal heart attack without warning.

Today's commercially sold sports drinks will not come close to replacing the necessary vitamins, amino acids, and 60 or more minerals required by strenuous sports. Most sports drinks contain only 2 minerals (sodium and potassium).

Sports drinks are big money enterprises. Just watch any sporting event on TV. Do you see the bottles and large coolers with the big "G" on the side? How about the sports managers squirting liquids into the athletes with the big "G" bottle during time outs? This is brilliant advertising by PepsiCo, the manufacturer of Gatorade. What about the classic Gatorade shower at the end of high profile football games? Even doctors recommend Gatorade to replace electrolytes when people are sick. Gatorade and Powerade contain sodium and potassium, that's it as far as minerals go. They also contain food colorings, sugars, and until recently, Gatorade and Powerade contained brominated vegetable oil (BVO) a flame retardant. Coca-cola has followed suit with Pepsico and is removing BVO from their drink products. I feel this is most likely due to consumer pressure. BVO has been replaced in Gatorade and Powerade and some soft drinks with esterified rosin. BVO and wood esters have been used as stabililzers to allow oil flavorings and carbonated water to exist in an emulsion (because oil and water do not mix). This rosin is esterified to reduce its allergy potential.(2) All BVO and esterified rosins have generally recognized as safe (GRAS) classification from the FDA. They are used to improve appearance and add absolutely no health or nutritional value to the product.

I vividly remember a Gatorade commercial showing green sweat coming from the pores of a very physical looking athlete. My reaction to that advertisement was- " *Wow! Look at the food colorings coming out of that guy!"*

Introducing Movement Properly

Let's look at a typical scenario that I often see in my office. A 275 lb. man comes in with hypertension, worn down knees, degenerative discs in his back, insomnia, skin problems, and fatigue. He wants to feel like he is 20 again; a pretty tall order. Where do we start?

First, we make sure that he is really invested in doing the program. I start exactly as described in the initial chapters. We get him to stop drinking man-made beverages and to start drinking pure water in proper amounts. Next on the agenda, is to eliminate wheat and all wheat products. Then we remove simple sugars, both refined and natural, including fruits. One half cup of blueberries, blackberries, raspberries or strawberries per day are allowed. Notice that I don't have him at the gym pumping iron and jogging on worn down arthritic knees while he is excessively overweight. We educate him on eating non-starchy carbs and quality cuts of free range meats in the proper amounts. He learns how important quality nutritious fats are to his overall health and function. He has learned why junk foods, food additives and hydrogenated trans-fats are so dangerous. We get him on the proper supplement program including essential vitamins, minerals, amino acids, and fatty acids.

I do not make him go to the gym and stress out his already stressed cardiovascular system or work out on arthritic knees, hips, or ankles.

After a couple of months he is losing weight and his nutrient stores are much improved (for some people this occurs more quickly). It is at this time I advise him to start walking, not a lot at first, but increasing every day by about ten or twenty steps. I tell him to park away from stores and walk a little further than he normally does. This is simple stuff. As he progresses, and continues to lose weight, he is also building his mineral reserves. I do not make him go to the gym and stress out his already stressed cardiovascular system or work out on arthritic knees, hips, or ankles. At the appropriate time, providing his cardiovascular capability is adequate (cleared by his physician), he can start "working out". This can be in the form of brisk walking, going to a gym, beginning a swimming program, and other activities. As he improves he can increase his intensity levels accordingly.

By this time we are several months into his transformation. We have made major dietary changes, nourished his body, and started with a "reasonable" level of physical activity. Our patient has adequate minerals, is properly hydrated, and the transformation is in full swing. Hopefully all parameters are improving. This patient is on the way to his long term goals and working to get off of his medicines with the help of his primary caregiver.

This is a typical case for someone that is obese and in poor overall health. While they are all uniquely different, the method is basically the same. There is some give and take as needed especially early in the program. My point is that exercise is not the initial key to success. Exercise becomes more important as the patient moves into a more healthy state. It's a process and there are usually years of poor eating and bad health habits that must be overcome. Stereotypes and emotional issues can add a lot of difficulty for some people. Those need to be worked through as well. When people really feel the changes occurring, the self-esteem begins to blossom. This is perhaps the most gratifying thing I see through a patients' transformation.

There are no quick fixes.

These things require time, understanding and dedication on the patient's part. There are no quick fixes. One of my patients told me "It was like eating an elephant it had to be done one bite at a time". I love that analysis. An old Chinese proverb says, "The journey of a thousand miles starts with one step." This is one of my favorite quotes to share with patients.

One thing that people absolutely need is hope. A lot of people have had their hopes dashed by their families, friends, or even their health care providers. This is sad but true. One of my diabetic REGENESIS program graduates told me that after years of programs that never worked, thousands of dollars and no results, and unmeasurable frustration, the most important thing is that this program gave her was hope. She continues to do well and is no longer considered diabetic by her doctors. She does not take any medications, she has lost over 125 lbs., and is under 140 lbs. for the first time in thirty years. She did not exercise in the beginning. She began walking gradually and now she is much lighter with normal health markers. Now she is walking about 2 miles a day. This will help her reach and maintain her long term goals.

I recently heard a quote I will paraphrase as I can't remember it exactly. "Aging does not cause you not to move, not moving causes you to age." There's a great deal of truth to that phrase. I have observed that a lot of aging patients are not so much losing strength as they are losing flexibility and mobility. One of the best exercises you can do if you are experiencing loss of flexibility and mobility is Tai Chi, the ancient Asian art of joint and muscle movement and light exercise. Tai Chi does not require a lot of strength and is not really a workout program, it's a movement program. It will make you move all of your joints through an active range of motion while increasing blood and lymphatic flow all over your body. It also helps to integrate left and right brain activity. DVD's on Tai Chi are readily available online.

I had a patient who was complaining about having difficulty getting up and out of his favorite chair. I gave him the simple exercise of getting up from of his chair 30 times a day. He had to get up and sit right back down 10 times and he was to do that 3 times a day. After one week he reported that he no longer had a problem getting up from his chair. This was a very simple solution; many solutions are just that simple. Others may be more complex and require a whole body approach to strengthening.

After initiating proper dietary changes and starting an adequate vitamin and mineral regimen is the best time to start exercising. Walking is my movement of choice in the early phases of a person's transformation. If you have a heart problem by all means consult with your heart doctor, or your general practitioner, to give you some guidance on what is an appropriate amount of exertion.

Another common problem that I often encounter is plantar fasciitis, a painful condition of the bottom of the feet. This occurs when the arches of the feet fall which can be brought about by excessive weight demands. Acute plantar fasciitis can occur with trauma and usually heals on its own. Chronic plantar fasciitis cannot be solved by exercise or surgery. It requires lifting the arches back into a more normal position. This is accomplished by the use of custom made orthotics. I use a company out of Roanoke VA. called Foot Levelers. I have great results with their products. If you have chronic plantar fasciitis, orthotics and an adjustment program from a good chiropractor, along with some myofascial release techniques are a must. Weight is a primary concern for chronic or severe plantar fasciitis. If the weight is not addressed, the problem cannot be totally corrected. I advise against foot surgeries or any other surgery unless they are absolutely necessary.

Do everything possible before consenting for painful surgery that requires lengthy recovery times. In short, if you have foot problems, exercise or movement becomes much more difficult, these problems must be resolved in order to move forward. The excess weight has to come off!

There are no strenuous exercises on the REGENESIS program as they are not necessary. My primary goal is to get a person to the place where they can take on a sport or high energy activity if they so desire. I want them to have the body, the health, and the nutritional understanding to do that. They could then take on a personal trainer, or another professional, to help them achieve their goals. Even with that being said, I still do not recommend high intensity exercises ever.

The benefits of exercise and other necessary movement is well documented and I don't want to create confusion here. It is extreme exercising without extreme nutrition that I am against. Reasonable exercise is very healthy for your heart, brain, and for prevention of diseases like diabetes, Alzheimer's disease, and cancer.

I certainly don't want you to think that I discourage exercising. I think a lot of people exercise who are not ready for the demands created by working out. Also, if you are malnourished, you may be doing more damage than good. Health is a multi-faceted thing, and working out can actually be dangerous if you are not in good nutritional health. From the book *God Bless America*:

> According to the CDC 100,000 young Americans under the age of 30 drop dead each year during or immediately following exercise or a game and that 300,000 Americans over the age of 30 drop dead annually during or after exercise. (3)

If you are into extreme conditioning or extreme sports, you had better be extremely nourished, especially with minerals. Initially, most of my patients are deficient in the requisite amounts of minerals needed for good health. I remember reading the account of Mark Sisson, a marathon runner, who wrote the book *Primal Blueprint*. He was a well-trained high intensity athlete. By the time he was in his 30's his body was broken down and wearing out. He discovered some basic simple truths about nutrition and literally rebuilt himself. At the printing of this book he is over 60 years old and in excellent condition. I am a big fan of his book and his recipes. The recipes and other information can be found at *marksdailyapple.com*. His book is also highly recommended. In it he chronicles the damage done to him by what he called "Conventional Wisdom" in regards to extreme conditioning. (4)

For good overall health, it's not necessary to do extreme physical workouts. Again, I suggest walking at first, some gentle beginner's yoga or Tai-Chi. As I mentioned previously, you must have made the necessary dietary changes and get a full complement of minerals, vitamins, amino acids, and essential fatty acids. As your health improves and your body adapts it is okay to increase intensity to a reasonable level. By this I mean increase your walking distance, join a gym and do mild to moderate weight training or go swimming. If you are new to the gym experience, I highly suggest hiring someone to help you get familiar with the equipment and help you do a beginner's exercise regimen. Most gyms have trainers who can help you. Spend a little money for some quality advice.

I do not recommend "carb loading" before you work out at the gym. Dr. Wallach always makes the point that, except for three baseball players from the old Negro Baseball League (1885-1951) [5], there has never been a professional athlete that has lived to be 100 years old. Extreme conditioning is not associated with a long life. Reasonable movement or mild to moderate exercise is. If extreme training created longevity football players would be a good representative sample of that. The Canadian Football League Players' Association reported,

> "..the average age for all pro football players, including all positions and back grounds, is 55 years. Several insurance carriers say it is 51 years." [6]

There is a lot of argument here. Dr. Wallach's premise: if conditioning alone created longevity, you would think that there would be a lot of 100 year old professional athletes around. This is a reasonable observation.

Hundred year old people have not spent a lot of time jogging, running marathons, or pumping iron at the gym.

11

Leftovers

*"As I see it, every day you do one of two things:
build health or create disease in yourself"*
Adelle Davis

I CALLED THIS chapter "Leftovers" because there were several things I wanted to address that did not warrant a chapter of their own. So the following few pages will be a hodgepodge of information designed to help you on your way to better health and hopefully answer some questions.

Goals

"Success is never final, failure is never fatal, and in discouragement is the word courage. It is courage that counts."
Winston Churchill

A very important thing to do when you are trying to do anything big is to set goals. Trying to recover your health is a big thing. It's bigger for some than others, but it still requires having goals. All of the big movers and shakers in business, and also motivational speakers, all across the board talk about setting goals. So there must be something to it, right? Ask anyone that is highly successful at anything and they will tell you they had goals, they wrote them down, and they looked at them frequently. I suggest you do the same.

I always make my patients set goals. Start with short term goals, and ultimately, a long term goal. Here is the kicker: When you reach your long term goal it is wise to set new goals for yourself. These goals are usually in some other area of your life. After you recover your health and vitality, all things are possible!!! New goals! New heights!! A dream or goal you once gave up on maybe worth reconsidering.

Write down three goals for yourself: Short, Medium and Long Term. While forming your goals, I want you to consider <u>why</u> you want to reach each one. This is very important. It's one thing to have a goal, but it's equally important why you want to reach that particular goal. Author John Locke says, *"Make your goals low enough to reach and high enough to matter"*. [1] After that is done, put your goals where you can see them. I suggest in the corner of the mirror where you get ready every day.

I ask my REGENESIS program participants to give me their goals and reasons. If they fall too far off the wagon, I will send them a copy of their goals with two questions: "What has changed?" and "How can I help you get back up?" It can be easy to lose focus. For some people it is just plain hard, especially if they have little or no support from their peer groups or family. I want my participants to know that I care about their progress. Sometimes, all it takes is just having someone in your corner. If there is someone you trust who knows you well, you may want to give them your goals. If they are doing the program too, perhaps you can swap goals. Accountability helps.

It's one thing to learn something it's another thing to put that knowledge to use. What are you willing to do with your new found knowledge? What are you willing to give up? If you are not willing to change, nothing will change for you. If you are unwilling to change setting goals will not work!!

Keep the mountain top in sight, keep your reasons close by, listen to people that will advance your knowledge, act on your new knowledge, continue to adapt, and stay on the program.

Attitude

> *"Accept that some day's you're the pigeon,*
> *and some days you're the statue."*
> Author unknown.

While it's not impossible, it's very difficult to help a person with a bad attitude about life and health. I have been able to plant some seeds of hope that did eventually take root. Those patients then moved on to make positive changes in their health and ultimately positive changes in their lives. I have spent some time on the negative side of life, and I can tell you from experience, the positive side is much better. I suffered from anxiety and panic attacks while I was in graduate school. The stress was great, our diets in school were pathetic, and we had what seemed to be little or no time to consider our own health. Looking back, I could have done a lot of things for my health I just didn't have the understanding at that time. That was a very difficult time for me and I was not thinking very positively. I just wanted to finish my education and get on with my life.

A good friend of mine saw the situation I was in and suggested the book *The Power of Now*, by Eckhart Tolle. (2) That one book changed the course of my life. I have since read so many books in that genre which have ultimately changed my view of the world and my place in it. I was fortunate to meet another one of my favorite authors, Dr. Wayne Dyer, at a conference in Las Vegas. I would also suggest any of his books to you. My favorite book by Dr. Dyer is *Your Erroneous Zones*. (3)

The point I want to make is that attitude matters as much, or maybe more, than anything else when it comes to your health journey. I remember a quote by Henry Ford who said, *"If you think you can do a thing, or think you can't do a thing, you're right."* Wow, is that ever true. If you start on a program that you are not emotionally invested in, and have no support, you are going to fail. On the flip side, if you are fully invested with the right attitude, and still have virtually no support, it's entirely possible to succeed. The important part of this combination is having the attitude that keeps you emotionally invested. You must truly want to change and your attitude must be in sync with your reasons to succeed. This is a winning combination.

Emotional Eating

"Life is about fulfillment."
Depak Chopra MD.

I know a lot of people who eat because of their emotions. Life has become very stressful for a lot of folks and eating is one of the few, possibly the only pleasure they may have. This leads to a downward spiral of obesity, poor health and disease that feeds the negative emotion. There are no simple answers for this for most people so I would like to suggest a good book to read as a starting point- *What Are You Hungry For* by Depak Chopra MD. In the book he says *"If your life isn't fulfilled, your stomach can never supply what's missing"*.[4] This is a difficult subject to take on and the book does a very good job of mapping out the problem and then how to deal with your emotions regarding foods. This book is very high on my reading list.

Stress

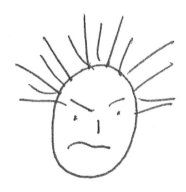

"I wear the chain I forged in life...I made it link by link, yard by yard"
Jacob Marley's character from *A Christmas Carol* by Charles Dickens

Stress is everywhere, it is unavoidable. Some people need stress for motivation, while others buckle under with minimal stress. When it comes to stress, people are all over the spectrum.

There are many kinds of stress. I use a very broad approach to this and focus on three kinds of stress: physical, chemical, and emotional. In the overall tally, your body doesn't know the difference, but the effects of all of these stressors is cumulative. We have talked about chemical stress in chapter 7 and there are chemical stressors in the SAD diet for sure. Emotional stress is highly variable from person to person, making it very hard to gauge. There is no "gold standard". Emotional eating occurs because people are lonely, unhappy in their lives, or have some unresolved conflict, like guilt or shame. If you do not deal with unresolved conflict, your life can become a contradiction, day after day after day. Physical stress is usually obvious: work, injury, repetitive motion, car wrecks, falls, etc. All stress causes some type of response from the body.

The fight or flight response is a genetic survival mechanism. This occurs in a primal part of your brain called the limbic system.(5) If primal man was threatened with bodily harm from something like being eaten by a tiger, his response was to either fight or run (flight). Today, if we feel stressed or threatened for any reason, the fight or flight response still kicks in. How much running or fighting do you do? The point here is that you carry stress around with you because we don't fight or run in response to stress anymore. We stick that stress somewhere inside of us and it accumulates over time. Over a period of days, weeks, or years, the effects of stress can manifest in sickness and poor health.

When people become stressed, it eventually takes its toll on the mitochondria (the energy producing part of every cell) and the adrenal glands (*ad-* means above, *renal* means kidney). These glands located on top of our kidneys are major players in the stress response. Mitochondrial disease is a new and emerging phenomenon that will be making its way into the headlines. Excess stress and the accompanying fatigue is a very common problem with patients. We can support mitochondrial function and the adrenals nutritionally, but in order to attain good health, the original stressors have to be removed or at least significantly reduced. It's impossible to remove all stress, but with some thought and action, stress can be successfully reduced.

There are countless ways to reduce stress. With the chemical variety you must first become aware of your exposure to chemicals. When possible you have to eliminate them from your life. From the previous chapters we know that most of the chemicals people are exposed to are in the home. Cleaning products, body care products, building materials, air fresheners, fabrics, and foods are the major culprits.

Physical stress varies from person to person. In a lot of cases it can be reduced with some effort. Improved ergonomics at work can help reduce physical stress. Better, more cautious, and deliberate movements at work can also help. Avoiding risky behavior should be obvious. For example, do not walk into oncoming traffic, operate machinery you know nothing about, or climb on ladders if you have little or no experience using ladders. A new and dangerous thing that people do is texting while driving. I saw a video of a woman who was looking at her text messages on her cell phone and fell into a pool like structure at the mall. A lot of our physical stress is caused by not paying attention, this is avoidable.

To discuss emotional stress adequately would require me writing several books. I often use the analogy that our lives are like movies. We are the director filming our own movie. We pick the actors, the location, and to a large degree, we direct the plot. Ultimately we can determine the length and quality of our movie if we avoid the pit falls of life. If you would like to read a good book on how to choose the characters in the movie that is your life, I would highly recommend the book *Boundaries* by Henry Cloud and John Townsend.[6] This book can help you to reduce the stress in your life caused by the people around you that seemingly do not respect you.

As you proceed through the REGENESIS program, your overall health should start to improve and you will be able to handle stress better, but it's still important to make yourself aware of your stressors. Awareness of why you eat the way you do is crucial for long term success. The more aware you become of your eating habits, the more you change your thoughts about food choices. This awareness along with knowledge and willpower is a recipe for a healthy outcome. Willpower is not enough on its own if you eat because of emotional needs. As I have discussed previously, knowledge alone is not adequate either. Knowledge coupled up with willingness and awareness will get you to where you want to be.

There are hundreds of books written on how to deal with stress. If you are having problems dealing with your particular stress, go to a book store, find a book, and then actually read it. If you dare, do some of the suggestions in the book! Bottom line, identify your stressors and deal with them. It will add quality years to your life.

Relax, Enjoy, Live

> *"Everyone chases after happiness,
> not noticing that happiness is right at their heels."*
> Bertolt Brecht

I often jokingly tell my patients, "It feels good to feel good." Of course it does. I say this because it's important to acknowledge when you feel good. It's easy to recognize, or remember, when you feel bad. Americans are so busy working, stressing, and worrying, that their lives often pass them by. When I have an unhappy patient in my office that is a workaholic or a real stress-head, I ask them this question, "What would you do if you had one or two days to live and you knew it?" I get some interesting answers. It never includes working more. It often involves spending more time with their loved ones, usually their children or grandchildren. I ask them the following questions: "If that is the case, then why aren't you doing that now?" and "Do you think you are going to live forever?" A great little book to read about this is *Who Will Cry When You Die,* by Robin Sharma.[7] He wrote another great fictional book called, *The Monk Who Sold His Ferrari.*[8] These are two great little books to read that could have a profound effect on how you view your life.

Slow down a little and take the time to relax more. When you take a vacation, go somewhere, don't stay home and paint the house. As the old saying goes, "stop and smell the roses". You shouldn't live to work, you should work to live. It's important to have a job that you like going to every day. If you hate your job, it's slowly killing you because of the emotional or physical stress it causes. It might be worth changing jobs even if it means taking a little less pay.

I love the work I do, but I need a break from it every once and a while. I need to enjoy the fruits of my labor from time to time. You don't have to go to Vegas or to Europe, just go somewhere and take a break. Vacations don't have to be costly. Plan for them, set aside a little money every week, and do it.

Meditation is a wonderful way to relax. It is also a good method of helping you deal with day to day stress. You can pick something that is troubling you and meditate about it. Meditation is an art form in and of itself, it requires some practice. There are a lot of good books and CD's available to help you learn how to practice meditation. One of my favorite authors, Wayne Dyer, states in his book *Getting in The Gap* (that also contains a meditation CD) that the average person has about 60,000 separate and often disconnected thoughts a day.(9) The reality is that most of us only need to have approximately 5000 or 6000 thoughts to navigate through one day. The rest of those thoughts are just "noise". Who needs that much noise in their lives? Learn how to cut out the noise using meditation and/or prayer.

Love and Forgiveness

"If God is the D.J., then Life is the dance floor.
Love is the rhythm and You are the music."
(unknown)

It is OK to love! Love comes in many forms and can be expressed in so many ways, from the grandiose to the simple. Love is a powerful emotion. I have found the greatest barrier to love is the inability to forgive. Forgiveness is often the precursor to being able to love. You must learn how to forgive others and to forgive yourself. You are not perfect and guess what, no one else is either. I know a lot of patients that are physically sick because they don't love themselves. They have not been able to forgive themselves or others in their lives. Often it's for things that happened years ago, and frequently for offenses unknown to the offender.

Many books have been written about love and forgiveness and the physical effects of repressed emotions. One of the books I read that had a profound effect on me was *Feelings Buried Alive Never Die,* by Carol

Truman. (10) Another great book by Wayne Dyer is, *There's A Spiritual Solution to Every Problem.*(11) If you are unable to forgive, love, or resolve emotional conflict, you can never attain optimal health.

And now these three remain: faith, hope, and love. But the greatest of these is love. 1 Corinthians 13:13

pH

> *"A healthy outside starts on the inside."*
> Robert Urich

This is a subject that has gained popularity over the last ten years. One of the premier books on the subject is *The pH Miracle* by Dr. Robert O. Young, and Shelley Redford Young.(12) The pH scale is an indicator of the concentration of hydrogen ions in solution. The most accepted definition of the abbreviation pH is "hydrogen potential". The scale runs from 1 to 14. Seven is considered neutral, one is highly acidic, and fourteen is highly alkaline (also called basic). Some chemistry classes are often called acid/base chemistry.

There are many things that influence the pH of the human body. Stress creates a very acidic body. A diet that is excessively high in protein can cause increased acidity. Smoking, food additives, and environmental chemicals can also tip the scale to the more acidic side. Being too acidic is called "acidosis".

Blood is slightly alkaline at around 7.36. It must stay very close to this range or the person will get very sick or even die. Saliva is generally neutral and the stomach is very acidic. The small intestine is generally alkaline at the beginning portion and much more acidic as it empties into the large intestine. The colon is acidic in the rectal area.

The Standard American Diet is very acidic. Junk foods, sugars, fried foods, excessive use of commercially produced red meats, wheat, soft drinks, and most bottled water are very acidic. Meats break down into amino "acids", therefore meats fall on the acidic side of the pH scale. Vegetables tend to be a lot more alkaline, especially the green leafy ones. Cucumbers for example are a very alkaline food. Barley grass and wheat grass are highly alkaline as well. Without getting too detailed on this complicated subject, it's wise to stay on the neutral to alkaline side of the scale if you want to be healthy. Alkalinity improves the absorption of minerals and vitamins. It helps fight infection and is very important in preventing and fighting certain kinds of cancers.

The REGENESIS program is alkalinizing and focuses on non-starchy carbohydrates as the foundation of the food part of the program. If you recall, I suggest several times through the preceding pages that you should eat fresh local non- starchy vegetables and, when you can, buy organic non GMO foods. Limit meat servings to the size of the palm of your hand (not The Jolly Green Giants' hand).

I highly recommend neutral or slightly alkaline water on this program. Bottled waters are usually highly acidic which is why there is an entire chapter devoted to drinking quality water. Make arrangements to carry your own water with you for the day in a proper vessel. Don't buy your water where you buy your soft drinks, candy bars, donuts, cigarettes, and gasoline. Hopefully after reading my book you will only use those places to buy gasoline.

If you stay on the REGENESIS program, you will be neutral to slightly alkaline. The REGENESIS program focuses on foods between 6 and 10 on the pH scale. An alkaline environment is also favorable for quality, consistent, sustainable weight loss. High protein diets keep you in ketosis which is very desirable for losing a lot of weight. For most people I don't feel that it's healthy to stay at high levels of ketosis for prolonged periods. This is especially true for people that are diabetic. Some patients with seizures and other conditions may respond well to a ketogenic diet. This diet can be difficult and hard to stay on long term because of limited food choices. There are exceptions to every diet. We are not all exactly the same.

You can measure your pH using pH test strips. According to Dr. Robert O. Young, ideal pH levels for morning saliva (before you brush your teeth or eat) is 7.2; for urinary pH the optimal level is 7.2 (2 hours after meals) [13] This takes a while to achieve if you have been eating the SAD diet. Not all acidic foods are bad. However, on average, Americans do too many things that create an acidic body. It's all about balance. Very few of my patients are "balanced" when they first come to my office as new patients.

...stress can make you very acidic very quickly.

If you continue to be acidic, it's usually due to stress, as stress can make you very acidic very quickly. When you stay in the acidic range for years, problems can develop. These problems include weight gain, allergies, food allergies, food intolerances, mood disorders, diabetes, osteoporosis, kidney problems, cancer, and fatigue. [14]

Cancer and pH is a frequently debated subject in holistic health care. I have read a lot about totally sugar free ketogenic diets (highly acidic) that starve cells of glucose, the primary fuel of cancer cells. I have also read a lot about highly alkaline vegetarian and juicing types of cancer diets that adhere more to the enzyme and anti-oxidant theories. Of particular curiosity to me here is the absence of processed sugars and rancid fats in both approaches. In the holistic approach, sugar and bad (rancid and hydrogenated) fats are absolutely enemy number one and two at each extreme and all points in the middle. I totally agree with the sugar free and bad fat free theories regarding cancer diets.

Many times I have heard the statement that cancer cannot grow in an alkaline environment. I have even said this myself. I am not so certain about this now as my knowledge about cancer is always evolving. Cancers come from improper DNA coding caused by nutritional deficiencies (especially minerals and amino acids), exposure to toxins, trauma, long term emotional stress factors, and unresolved conflict, not merely the lack of an alkaline environment.

If you have cancer, dietary changes are essential to your survival, do some research and chose your plan carefully. Most traditional cancer doctors place little to no importance on diet, this is a big problem. I recently watched a local cancer doctor on our hometown news channel. He was answering some of the most common questions about cancer.

pH of some common foods
Alkaline 14

- 10   Wheatgrass, Barley grass, Cucumbers, Broccoli, Artichokes, Onion, Cabbage, Kale, Lemon, Lime
Avocado, Green Tea, Sweet Potatoes, Green Beans, Blueberries, Beets
- 9   Eggplant, Squash, Lettuce, Cauliflower, Spinach
- 8   Grapefruit, Tomatoes, Mushrooms, Peppers, Strawberries, Radishes, Olives.

Neutral 7   Tap water, Spring Water, River Water, Municipal Water

- 6   Fruit Juices, Grains, Eggs, Salmon, Coconut, Brown Rice, Barley, Oats
most meats.
- 5   Bottled Waters, pastries, donuts, candies, pizza dough.
- 4   Pasta, Popcorn, Chocolate, Black Tea, Beer, Wine, Soft Drinks, Energy
- 3   drinks

Acidic 1

One of the questions from a viewer was (I am paraphrasing) – *"Does sugar feed cancer?"* His response was an immediate and stern "<u>NO</u>". Don't count on traditional oncologists to give you adequate nutritional advice. As you recall, I mentioned previously that one of my patients who has a husband with cancer, was offered Cokes and donuts at one of their oncology visits.

I don't really have a "bottom line" on pH but I do lean towards an alkaline diet and lifestyle. Following the REGENESIS program will most likely put you into the slightly alkaline range providing your stress levels are low. Again, there are some people that do very well on diets in the acidic range providing they are eating quality foods. I am a proponent of ketogenic diets for some people. People that suffer from seizures, polycystic ovarian syndrome, and a few other conditions can do very well on an adequately designed ketogenic program.

Free Radicals and ORAC points

Free radicals are defined as "atoms, ions or molecules with unpaired electrons or an open shell configuration."[15] Free radicals have negative, positive or zero charge. With some exceptions, these unpaired electrons cause radicals to be highly chemically "reactive". Without getting into an organic chemistry lecture here, let me just say that free radicals exist in everyone. Some free radicals, such as the ones used in redox signaling (biological messengers), are actually very beneficial and essential to good health. It's when harmful free radical consumption or production overtakes the ability of the body to counter them that trouble begins. One of the most common sources of free radicals in humans is rancid fats.

The body balances or overcomes free radicals with antioxidants that are found in foods like brightly colored fruits and vegetables. Vitamin A, vitamin C, vitamin E, and selenium (ACES) are antioxidants. Excessive free radical consumption and production, unchecked by a lack of antioxidants, accelerates the aging and the disease processes in humans. Stress, alcohol, poor diet, food chemicals, rancid fats, and smoking are major causes of free radicals.

A diet that is high in quality antioxidants free from rancid fats and foods with chemical additives that create free radicals, is essential for good health. Locally grown organic vegetables and fruits are good sources of natural antioxidants. The REGENESIS program encourages the consumption of colorful non-starchy vegetables, above all other food choices. The supplement that I generally recommend is loaded in antioxidants from 115 fruits, vegetables and super juices. (The supplements that I recommend can be found at the website www.regenesis4health.com).

I also recommend quercetin, resveratrol, and turmeric, three very powerful antioxidants. Quercetin in particular is a very powerful anti-cancer nutrient and a natural anti-histamine. It is found in high concentrations in muscadine grape seeds and apple skins. Resveratrol is also found in muscadine grapes as well as other grapes, raspberries, blueberries and pomegranates. Tumeric is a yellow spice that comes from a plant in the ginger family. It grows in southern Asia and requires a lot of rainfall. It's also found in curry, a popular Indian seasoning.

General health recommendations vary from 3,000 to 25,000 ORAC points a day. The REGENESIS program will provide adequate oxygen radical absorbance capacity (ORAC) points a day if you are adequately supplementing and eating a full complement of colorful veggies and berries. It is worth mentioning that cultures with a history of living long lives consume greater amounts of antioxidants in natural forms [16].

A lot of chemotherapy drugs deliberately create free radicals in the body. Cancer doctors often tell people not to take vitamins, especially Vitamin C, folic acid, and others, during chemotherapy. I feel it is necessary to mention that a 2006 oncology study reveals that cytotoxic (toxic to cells) chemotherapy for <u>malignant</u> cancers has a 5 year success rate of less than 3%. That means it has a 97% failure rate! Realistically, chemotherapy is only effective in improving five year survival rates in a few common cancers including Hodgkin's disease (35.8%) and testicular cancer (41.8%) according to the study. [17] Why do we use this toxic approach so much? My guess is because it is highly profitable and cancer is such a frightening diagnosis. More and more people are rejecting chemotherapy for natural health options. Some people are incorporating both. These decisions are very difficult and personal. I do not know anyone who has not lost loved ones to cancer.

Milk

"Never cry over spilt milk, because it may have been poisoned."
W.C. Fields

Milk for some reason, has become controversial. Humans have been drinking raw milk from cows and goats (and raw breast milk from humans) for thousands of years. I don't want to spend too much time here as there could be volumes written about this. I will point you to a good source on the subject of raw milk: www.realmilk.com. There is a wealth of information at this website. Weston A. Price foundation also has a lot of information regarding raw (whole) milk.

I grew up on raw milk in our rural setting in southwest Virginia. I can still remember the smell of wild pasture onion grass in the milk from time to time. One of our neighbors would churn butter from the rich cream, it was more than delicious. As far as I know many of the families that lived near us also used raw milk, I never knew of any of them that ever got sick from it. As a matter of fact, as children we rarely ever got sick period. We played in the creeks, handled bugs and animals of all sorts, and yes we drank raw milk.

The FDA claims that "Raw milk can harbor dangerous micro-organisms that can pose serious health risks to you and your family".[18] The rebuttal to this comment by RealMilk.com is as follows-

It is possible for raw milk to harbor dangerous micro-organisms, but it is possible for ANY food, raw or pasteurized, to harbor dangerous micro-organisms. We do not advocate drinking unpasteurized milk from modern Holsteins, bred to produce high volumes of milk, injected with recombinant Bovine Growth Hormone (rBGH), and raised in commercial feedlots where they are crowded and stressed and given antibiotics to keep them from being sick. That milk DOES need to be pasteurized to lessen (not eliminate) the possibility of food-borne illness. We advocate the drinking of raw milk from old-fashioned breeds of cows raised on pasture, with plenty of green grass, sunshine, and room to move. Properly raised and milked in clean conditions, this milk is extremely unlikely to harbor dangerous micro-organisms...in fact, less likely than commercial, pasteurized milk. (19)

We seem to have this idea that if milk is pasteurized that it is naturally safe. Think again. Quoting again from the RealMilk article-

...when consumers become ill from pasteurized commercial milk, hundreds or thousands are often sickened. The largest outbreak of food-borne illness from pasteurized milk occurred in March of 1985 when there were 19,660 confirmed cases of Salmonilla typhimurium illness FROM CONSUMING PROPERLY PASTERUIZED MILK. Pasteurization is no guarantee of milk safety, and in fact, raw milk destined for pasteurization is allowed to have more bacteria in it both before and after pasteurization than raw milk that is destined to be consumed raw. (20)

The machines used for pasteurization also pose a problem. Milk is shipped in tanker like trucks to the milk processing factories. There it passes through long pipes as it is put through different high-temperature processes. These pipes and the tanker trucks must be regularly cleaned using industrial cleaners and solvents. The residues of these solvents end up in the finished product. This is only one of many reasons I am an advocate for quality raw milk and butter. (21)

Besides the chemical problem, pasteurization destroys natural milk enzymes, creates rancidity in the unsaturated milk fats, decreases availability of the mineral components like calcium and magnesium, and denatures the milk proteins.(22)

Got Milk? Yes I do, but personally, mine will be raw thank you. Do your research here if you insist on using milk, make an educated choice for you and or your family. Some states allow the purchase of raw milk, in other states you must own a "share" of a cow in order to consume raw milk. It is amazing to me that here in Virginia, I can buy alcohol that is responsible (directly and indirectly) for a lot of deaths, but I cannot buy healthy raw milk like I drank for over 20 years of my life. I do not allow processed milk (whole, 2%, 1%, or skim) on the REGENESIS program. I will allow quality cheese (available in any state) on the program. Do not eat imitation cheese products!

Food Labels

"Cooking is not chemistry, it is art. It requires instinct and taste rather than exact measurements."
Marcel Boulestin

It is very important to know how to read food labels. I am always amazed by how little people know about this. While preparing for some of my REGENESIS classes, I copied the food labels of three commonly consumed items. I presented them using a power point presentation. Almost everyone in the classes missed the basic questions I asked regarding simple analysis of the labels. Questions about serving size were missed by everyone. Most of the classes did not understand the labeling of carbohydrates/sugars.

I want you to look at what you are buying and consuming. It is required by law to label foods. I personally feel that labeling should be more strict, but we must learn to play the cards we have. Let's look at two food labels and navigate through what they tell us.

Food label #1

A generic biscuit mix label

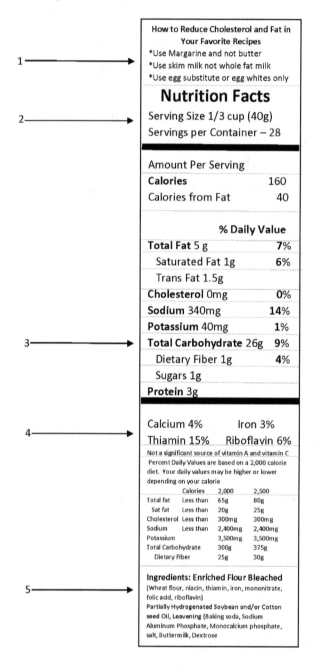

1. From food label #1, the cooking instructions recommend using margarine, skim milk, and egg substitutes in order to reduce fat and cholesterol.

2. Look at the serving size, there are 28 servings per box. The serving size is very important. Most soft drinks are 2 or 2-1/2 servings per container. If you are monitoring your carb consumption, you must multiply total carbs by the number of servings you are going to consume. In this case a serving is 1/3 of a cup (a biscuit I presume). 1/3 of a cup has 26 grams of carbs.

3. Look at the total carbohydrates, 26 g. per serving (1 biscuit). If you have 2 biscuits, you will have consumed 52 grams of carbs! There are 728 total grams of carbohydrates in the entire box of mix. If 1 teaspoon contains 4 grams of sugar, that equals 91 teaspoons of carbohydrates in the entire box.

4. This box contains the basic vitamin and mineral contents per serving. Keep in mind a lot of wheat products are "enriched". This means the vitamins have been added back after the manufacturing process. A lot of the vitamins used in this "enrichment" are synthetic. If a food is nutritious from nature, it shouldn't have to be enriched. This happens because the wheat is refined and stripped of most of the beneficial nutrients.

5. This is the ingredient list. It is listed in descending order. The first listed item is the most plentiful, the second ingredient is the second most plentiful, and so on.

Notice in this product there is **Enriched Flour Bleached** (wheat flour). Also there is **partially hydrogenated soybean and/or cottonseed oil**. We previously covered the dangers of these oils extensively. Avoid anything that has hydrogenated fats of any kind.

Food Label #1 comes from a typical biscuit mix. This product can also be used to make various wheat containing foods from pie crust, pancakes, and fried chicken. In typical grocery stores, there is often a huge section in the baking aisle isle devoted to very popular products like this. They are convenient to use and inexpensive. Products like this are often made with highly hybridized wheat, hydrogenated fats, and preservatives. Egg substitutes and margarine recommended on this label are very unhealthy foods. I am always amused that there are reduced cholesterol instructions on some of these products. It is the use of these highly refined carbohydrate grains in products like this that can cause the very inflammation responsible for elevating cholesterol levels.

The next label (food label #2) is an example of a pot roast TV dinner. I have briefly discussed TV dinners in general and how toxic they are by my standard. They are generally loaded with hydrolyzed, autolyzed, modified starch products, highly processed oils, preservatives, and other additives that are nowhere close to "natural". Does anyone want to guess what "modified food starch" products are? Companies are aware that consumers are reading labels and trying to avoid MSG, so they cleverly use another name like hydrolyzed protein to disguise the fact that their products contain a great deal of this neurotoxin. TV dinners and boxed pizzas have strikingly similar ingredients. Most boxed microwavable commercial products contain MSG as well as a plethora of unhealthy additives. None of the products mentioned above are allowed on the REGENESIS program.

These products are completely legal and all of the additives and ingredients are deemed safe by the FDA. TV dinners and boxed pizzas are a large segment of the foods purchased in America. I am entitled to my opinion based on my knowledge and I personally feel that most of these products are very unhealthy.

There is an emerging market for healthier TV dinners. There are organic and some gluten free selections of TV dinners and soups. I have listed acceptable products on regenesis4health.com. Use them sparingly.

TV Dinners (food label#2)

Flavoring (MSG?) Natural Flavoring (MSG?) Hydrolyzed proteins (excitotoxins)

> **INGRDIENTS: SAUCE** (WATER, BURGUNDY WINE, SALT) MODIFIED CORNSTARCH, TOMAO PUREE, BEEF BASE [ROASTED BEEF AND CONCENTRATED BEEF STOCK, HYDROLYZED (CORN GLUTEN, SOY, CORN AND WHEAT) PROTEIN, CORN OIL, SUGAR, CORN MALTODEXTRIN, YEAST EXTRACT, CARMEL COLOR, FLAVORING, SALT], NATURAL FLAVORING, BEEF FAT, REDUCED LACTOSE WHEY AND WHEY (MILK), CORN STARCH, SUGAR, SALT, MODIFIED CORNSTARCH, POTATO STARCH, BEET POWDER, LIPOLYZED CREAM, CORN SYRUP SOLIDS, DISODIUM GUANYLATE, SALT, ROASTED BEEF TYPE FLAVOR [YEAST EXTRACT], SOY SAUCE (WATER SOYBEANS, WHEAT, SALT), FLAVORING, SUGAR, FLAVOR ENHANCER (DEXTROSE, SALY, AUTOLYZED YEAST EXTRACT, MODIFIED CORN STARCH], CARAMEL COLOR [CONTAINS SULFITES], XANTHAN GUM, RED WINE VINEGAR, SUGAR. **FULLY COOKED SEASONED BRAISED BEEF POR TOAST DICES AND MODIFIED FOOD STARCH PRODUCT** (BEEF, WATER, WITH 1.5%DEXTROSE, SALT, MODIFIED CORNSTARCH, CONCENTRATED BEEF STOCK, SODIUM PHOSPHATES, POTASSIUM CHLORIDE, CARAMEL COLOR, SPICE EXTRACTIVES), **CARROTS, ONIONS, ROASTED RED POTATOES. GREEN BEANS.**CONTAINS. MILK. WHEAT. SOY

Corn Syrup (GMO Corn?)   Modified Food starch (MSG?)   Modified Corn Starch (MSG?)

Radical?

I have had several patients and class participants tell me that my plan was too "radical" for them. I just want to touch on that before you turn the page to the dietary part of my program. As you have read in the body of this book, I suggest drinking pure water as you were meant to, eating non-starchy healthy vegetables, consuming reasonable portions of meats, avoiding man-made chemicals (including medicines), reducing your consumption of sugars and grains and taking supplements to ensure that your body is adequately nourished. I don't feel that this is "radical".

I do have an opinion on what I feel <u>IS</u> "radical". Consuming dead, sugar laden, chemically altered foods is "radical". Taking 5, 6, or 15 prescription drugs is "radical". Having 3 - 5 doctors is "radical". Living on fast foods and soft drinks especially diet drinks is "radical". Weighing 275 to 350 or even 400 lbs. is "radical". Having to have joint replacements because you have been overweight for 40 years is "radical". Living for 10 years in a nursing home because you chose not to take good care of your health is "radical". Making healthy people pay for the excessive health care needs of people that have knowingly made poor decisions in their lives is "radical". Being in the sickest, most overweight, most prescription drug consuming nation in the world is "radical".

I know this may sound cruel to some people, however it is the truth as I see it. I don't play softball with my patients. They have already had that from their doctors, families, friends, and governmental agencies. Our generous society has always taken care of the people that truly could not care for themselves. I understand that a portion of the population truly could not have prevented or changed their health status. However, this is the exception more than the rule. I have deep sympathy for those people and I absolutely want a portion of my tax dollars to go to their needs. I donate my time and talents to patients that truly cannot afford my services. I donate money and participate in local fund raisers and encourage my staff and patients to do the same. These things are best taken care of on a local level most of the time.

If you are radically sick and unhealthy, it will take what seems to be "radical" changes to correct that. Eating in a healthy manner, reading health books, eliminating chemicals, drinking pure water, and taking responsibility for your health is not "radical". Now, my "radical" ranting is over.

In Summary

In summary, check your pH, set your goals, learn how to read food labels, adjust your attitude, work on your stressors, relax, live, practice forgiveness, and love! Meditate, pray. Oh yea, and for goodness sake, take a vacation once in a while!

12

Eating Guidelines

"Unfortunately, man is the victim of his appetites."
Norman Walker

THE REGENESIS DIETARY recommendations are balanced. It is not low fat, low or no carbohydrate diet, it's not high in protein. Ancient Chinese teachings are replete with the concepts of "balance", and "nothing to excess". The dietary recommendations found in the following pages are balanced and there is no excess.

I have deliberately chosen to do the eating guideline in a different style. Many folks will buy a health or diet book and go directly to the diet part to see what is allowed. They will not take the time to actually read the why and why not parts of the program in the bulk of the book. This way the reader has to read these guidelines, not just a food list. The food guidelines and suggestions are scattered all over the place so please read on.

This guideline is steeped in trial and error as well as common sense. It works because it is a natural way to eat. It is from God's bounty placed here specifically for our nutritional needs. The closer a food is to its natural form the better, the fewer additives the better, the less man has to do with it the better! As my understanding and education moves forward, there may be more additions, or even subtractions, from this guideline. Just like the reader, my knowledge base is constantly changing and evolving.

PHASE 1

Let's start the guideline by saying: Non-starchy vegetables are preferred to all other foods. Meats and eggs are totally acceptable but free range is preferred. If you are a vegetarian, that is fine too. Pay particular attention to the allowable oils as this is crucial to good health.

You must eliminate all processed meats including deli meats. This also includes bologna, hot dogs, souse meats, spam, treet, and potted meats. Avoid canned ham, tuna, and chicken. These meats contain nitrites, nitrates, and other additives. Nitrite and nitrate free bacon, sausage, and other meats can be purchased at most health food stores and some of the large chain stores.

Nitrites when heated create substances called nitrosamines which have been scientifically proven to be highly carcinogenic. Beef, bison, pork, and chicken should be free range and free of antibiotics. Free range wild meats are acceptable if they are slaughtered and prepared properly. Meat portions should not be any larger than the palm of your hand for each meal. If you really like hot dogs, I suggest Applegate brand which are allowed on this program. They are all-natural, organic, free range, nitrite and nitrate free, and can be found at most health food stores. Small amounts of nitrites occur naturally in some meats. It is the additional nitrites and nitrates that are problematic.

Never eat burned or seared meats! You are asking for trouble down the line when the cancer from the nitrosamines and heterocyclic amines shows up. Meats are best prepared by baking, broiling, or stewing. Learn how to use a crock pot. People of Scandinavian descent that live in the upper midwest outlive southerners by 10 -15 years. What do they do differently? They rarely fry foods and they eat soups and stews all the time. If you like to use the BBQ grill, learn how not to burn your meats.

Fish, preferably wild caught, is another good source of protein and essential fatty acids and should be included frequently. A great place to buy quality, wild caught, BPA free, canned Alaskan salmon is from a company called *Vital Choice* (I have a link to their website at regenesis4health.com). Fresh seafood (not farm raised) is acceptable. Do not eat breaded shrimp, clams or fish or fish "sticks".

Starchy carbohydrates are not allowed on the program. This includes white and red potatoes. Potatoes will spike your blood sugar as fast as a spoonful of white sugar! Also, not allowed are common beans including pinto, Octobers, lima beans, garbanzo beans, hummus, red beans, pork n' beans, kidney beans, and others. Green beans are allowed and are a highly preferred food. Peanuts and peanut butter are not allowed. Peanuts are really beans (legumes) and are high in aflatoxins (naturally occurring fungal toxins), this is why they stopped serving them on airplanes. A small exception I will make here is lentils. I like the amino acid content of organic lentils so one small serving (1 cup) or a serving of lentil soup is allowed if it is the only carbohydrate of the meal. Lentils fall short of delivering all the amino acids by one, methionine which is found in eggs, fish, and meat products.

Non-starchy vegetables are my favorite and preferred foods. Among them are all the green leafy vegetables, eggplant, cucumbers, and squash of all kinds. More and more squash is being genetically modified so buy them organically if possible. Sweet potatoes are allowed and are another one of my favorites. Eat them often with butter and cinnamon for one of nature's treats, and yes I am aware that it is not exactly a non-starchy carb. Sweet potatoes are loaded in vitamin A and other beneficial nutrients. Peppers of all kinds are allowed, as are onions, leeks, celery, Swiss chard, carrots, and mushrooms. Olives, asparagus, artichokes, avocados, and tomatoes are also allowed and are preferred foods. Frozen vegetables are a better choice than canned vegetables. Fresh in season and local vegetables are always preferred.

Cruciferous vegetables are allowed on the plan as they have many health benefits. The most common ones include broccoli, cauliflower, brussels sprouts, cabbage, kale, mustard greens, kohlrabi, watercress, bok-choy, and horseradish. However, IF YOU HAVE THYROID ISSUES, cruciferous vegetables can inhibit thyroid function and should be avoided.

ALL WHEAT PRODUCTS MUST BE AVOIDED!! I'm on cap locks here because I am screaming that I do not want you to eat any wheat products. Wheat is one of the carbohydrates notoriously hidden in other foods like soup. I devoted an entire chapter to wheat. It will raise and keep your blood sugar levels high, not to mention that it is one of the unhealthiest foods ever created. Yes, today's wheat has been created by scientists. If you don't believe me, then you have not read the book *Wheat Belly*. I highly suggest you read it. No biscuits, breads, cereals, donuts, pretzels, pancakes, waffles, cakes, pies cookies, gravies, pasta noodles, or anything that contains wheat. Do not use bread substitutes as they will raise blood sugar levels just as much as wheat breads.

Rice is an acceptable grain if it is whole grain rice in small portions and is the only carbohydrate with the meal. White rice is not included. Rice pasta noodles can be used as a substitute in pasta dishes. However, be aware of the carbohydrate content of this food. Remember we are trying to keep blood sugar levels low and steady. When you are eating Chinese foods (MSG free of course) do not eat a plate full of rice.

No cereals are allowed! Cereals are high in carbohydrates. Most cereals are super-heated and some are forced through a high pressure extruder. They may contain acrylamides and are loaded with carbohydrates and added sugars. Do not start your day off with carbohydrates! You will crave carbs all day if you do. Start your day with protein and quality fat, like eggs and nitrite-free breakfast meats. Try something different and eat eggs with a sweet potato. Don't be afraid to try different foods for breakfast!

Corn, barley, rye, and oatmeal are not permitted. Steel-cut oats are allowed, but only in small portions (1 cup cooked). No popcorn, as this is a superheated carbohydrate and when you superheat carbs, you create acrylamides that are suspect in causing cancer!

Absolutely no vegetable oils are allowed. For example: Wesson oil, Crisco, soy oil, canola oil, cottonseed oils, or corn oils. None of the so called heart-healthy hydrogenated spreads are allowed. Absolutely no margarine should be used because of hydrogenation and other steps used in manufacturing them. They are also very high in poor quality Omega 6 oils.

Acceptable for cooking are real butter, lard (yes, lard), and free range beef tallow. Try to limit, and eventually eliminate, frying as a means of cooking foods. Olive oil can be used as salad dressing only. Buy small bottles of cold pressed extra virgin olive oil and keep it in a cool dark location. Olive oil will go rancid over time. It is best to <u>avoid all oils</u> in the long run. Learn to eat without them, use lemon or lime juice over your salads (the taste will surprise you). Coconut oil is a super food and is okay if it is purchased in small bottles, stored appropriately and used in a short time span.

Eggs are totally acceptable on this program if you are not allergic to them. The preferred cooking method is poached, followed by boiled. If you want to fry them, do so lightly in butter over low heat. Free range eggs are rich in organic sulfur (onions, garlic and leeks are also rich in sulfur).

It has been my experience that most people are sulfur deficient. We have already discussed how the sulfur cycle was broken in 1954 when nitrogen based chemical fertilizers were being used instead of sulfate based fertilizers. These chemicals lack the bioavailability of natural minerals. Your body does not store sulfur so it must be consumed daily, and eggs are a great source of this vital mineral. Do not confuse sulfur with sulfa drugs, they are not the same. Many people have been injured or killed by sulfa drugs. This mistakenly makes some people afraid of anything with the ingredient sulfur. If you have a problem with eggs, garlic, and onions, you may have a sensitivity to sulfur containing foods and supplements.

Eggs do contain cholesterol, but you need high quality cholesterol in your diet. Eating quality cholesterol does not cause your blood cholesterol to elevate. I will say this again, *stress, eating junk food, rancid oils, and sugars make your cholesterol go up!* Do not be afraid of eating true FREE RANGE eggs, they are packed full of good nutrition. I do not trust the quality of commercially produced eggs and do not approve of the unsanitary and crowded conditions in which these animals live. Find a good local farmer or egg producer that captures eggs from free ranging hens.

Berries are allowed: blueberries, raspberries, and strawberries. Be aware that strawberries greatly absorb chemicals used in the growing process. So, the only strawberries allowed are those that are organically grown and not sprayed with pesticides. A small handful of organic cherries of any kind are allowed when they are in season.

I do not allow other fruits on the program because of their high simple sugar content. I am deliberately trying to keep the daily insulin production low. No fruit juices or dried fruit for the same reasoning, it causes a spike in insulin. Some fruits may be introduced during phase 2 of the program.

White sugar, or any other kind of sugar like turbinado or raw sugar, is not allowed on this program! Honey is not allowed, neither are maple syrup, date sugar, and agave. Stevia drops are the only allowed sweetener. Quality stevia is hard to find and usually has to be purchased at health food stores. Look for stevia drops because they are not loaded with other additives. Lemon water seems to help curb sugar cravings, so use lemons or limes in your water. Make lemonade or limeade by using lemon water and stevia drops (very tasty).

The only time you can have any sugar is if you are diabetic and your blood sugar levels "crash", then for obvious reasons do what you have to do. After being on the program for a while, your insulin levels should become very steady and "crashing" is something that should not happen. Infection, stress, erratic eating habits, and certain medications can cause broad fluctuations in blood sugar levels. These issues are best addressed by you and your physician.

The use of artificial sweeteners is not allowed on the REGENESIS program. I am speaking here in particular about Splenda (sucralose), Nutra Sweet (Aspartame), and Acesulfame-K. These sweeteners cause you to have food cravings. I personally think they are some of the most dangerous food additives in America. No matter what you have heard or read about the safety of artificial sweeteners, if you have read what I have suggested, you will never consume them again because you will know what I know. Also, avoid sugar alcohols (mannitol, sorbitol, xylitol, isomalt, and erythritol).

Do not drink soft drinks, ever. Give them up. No Kool-Aid, Gatorade, Powerade, sports drinks like AMP, Monster and Red Bull. Rebound FX from *Youngevity*, is a good sports drink and is allowed on the REGENESIS program. Learn to drink quality water as it's what you were meant to drink. When a deer needs something to drink, it does not go into a convenience store and buy a soda or a sports drink, it goes to the creek and drinks water. Deer and other creatures know where to find water. I suggest you learn where to find good water and drink it often. Owners freak out when they see their dog drinking from a mud puddle. Our pets are instinctively drawn to muddy water for its mineral content. But man, in all his wisdom, has poisoned the planet. Our mud puddles are now laced with petroleum and chemical runoff. While it was once okay for dogs to drink from mud puddles, I don't let my pets drink from puddles anymore.

The use of coffee was discussed in the chapter on water. Coffee has a considerable dehydrating effect. It also competes to some degree with absorption of minerals. Most Americans are grossly mineral deficient. If you must drink coffee, drink an antioxidant coffee, I suggest *Jafa Fit* from *Youngevity* (see regenesis4health.com). Drink only one cup at least one hour before or after you take your minerals. For every cup of coffee you drink, you should drink two equivalent cups of water to remain hydrated.

<u>Mild</u> herbal teas are acceptable. Green tea is acceptable as long as it is not your only source of liquids. It is optimal to avoid all alcoholic beverages and this is imperative if you are a diabetic. Alcohol is a pure carbohydrate and will spike your blood sugars. An <u>occasional</u> glass of wine (dark red) or a wheat free beer (like Red Bridge) is acceptable. Be sure to factor the carbohydrate content of these beverages into your daily carbohydrate consumption. It needs to be between 50 and 100 grams per day depending on your weight.

Foods that come through your car window are not allowed. Commercial and boxed pizzas are not allowed. If you can't pronounce it on the label, do not eat it. TV dinners are not allowed. Read the ingredients on a TV dinner, they are crazy. Right after you read the label, if it is in your house, throw it in the trash!

No bouillon or food product that involves or contains a "flavor packet", such as various hamburger flavorings, flavored noodles, and some pre-packaged flavored rice dishes. Most of these flavor packets are loaded with MSG and other garbage. If you want to use soup stock like vegetable or chicken broth, read the labels. Make sure there is no MSG or spices that contain MSG, or hydrolyzed vegetable protein. Remember from chapter 6 that there are many names for MSG.

One of the problems with going on a new food program designed to reduce insulin is that it limits carbs. In many people, the cravings for something sweet seem to persist. I personally love chocolate and I have discovered that if you develop a taste for dark chocolate (no milk chocolate or artificial sweeteners) and only do one or two little squares of it a day, this makes an acceptable treat. It must be over 70% <u>organic</u> dark chocolate and only one or two small squares per day! Don't go overboard here. One bar should last you almost a week. If you find yourself eating more than that, stop buying it and don't have it in the house to tempt you. I'm trying to allow something here to get you to stay on the program and not feel deprived of a simple treat. I'm giving a couple of inches, don't take a mile.

As a rule, canned soups are not acceptable on the program for several reasons. They often contain wheat, MSG, hydrolyzed proteins and other chemicals including BPA from the can liners. So, don't eat canned soups or any other canned products (BPA free organic canned foods are allowed). For vegetables, if the decision is over canned or frozen, chose frozen and organic if it is available. There are a few companies that are starting to use BPA free cans. This market is evolving, so keep looking online for companies that are changing. There are companies that make organic canned beans in BPA free cans like Eden Organic, and Amy's. I allow their products on the program. However, I always prefer fresh over canned foods.

When you go out to eat, drink water and order salads, steamed veggies, and small portions of meat. It is appropriate to ask if it is tap water or filtered water, the wait staff should know. If it is only tap water, opt for glass bottled water if it is offered. Pass on the dessert.

Do not preach at the people you are eating with about their food choices. Enjoy yourself and the company of your friends and loved ones. Live by example. It took me years to figure out not to lecture people when we are eating out, especially if they really didn't ask for my advice. I was doing it out of concern but that is not always the way it was perceived.

Many sauces, dips, and dressings used at restaurants contain MSG. It pays to know which restaurants use these products and to avoid eating there. For example, the salsas at some Mexican restaurants have MSG in them. Most Chinese eateries use MSG.

If you do not have an allergy to dairy, eating cheese is okay, but do not eat imitation cheese. Quality cheese is a protein rich food source and certainly adds to the eating experience. Raw milk is okay if it is from a reputable source. Processed milk is not allowed (no 1%, 2%, skim milk, or whole milk). If you live in a state like Pennsylvania that allows the sale of raw milk, I am jealous of you. Once milk is pasteurized and homogenized, it is no longer milk and becomes a highly processed and unhealthy food. Yogurt is acceptable if it is organic and not one filled with sugar and fruit. MSG has found its way into yogurt now and is often called "natural flavoring", avoid these brands. Do not eat light yogurt as it contains artificial sweeteners. Eat plain yogurt and add to it some of the acceptable berries and stevia drops to sweeten it if desired. The active cultures in the yogurt are good for your intestines. I suggest you eat real butter (pure raw from whole milk). Don't eat it like a popsicle, but it is okay to use in moderation. Buy quality butter or ghee, raw free range butter from a reputable source is best if you can find it. DO NOT EAT MARGARINES, COOL WHIP, OR USE POWDERED COFFEE CREAMERS!!!!

Do not eat potato chips, cheese puffs, deep fried corn products, pork rinds, or chips that all have exactly the same shape. Think about it, chips that all have exactly the same shape have to be a totally fabricated "food".

Nuts are acceptable with a little understanding. Peanuts are not nuts. Again, they are not allowed on the REGENESIS program. Nuts are best if they are raw and organic, roasted is okay, soaked and or sprouted are preferred. Acceptable nuts are walnuts, cashews, pecans, pistachios, almonds, Brazil nuts, and macadamia nuts. I personally purchase my nut butters and sprouted nuts from Blue Mountain Organics. Nuts are great for in-between meal snacks. Only eat about a handful at a time. Do not eat canned nuts if they contain cottonseed oils. Nut butters are acceptable if they are good quality. Nuts are a good source of essential oils and have a lot of good qualities. For example, almonds have some anti-cancer properties and walnuts are good at preventing certain parasites.

Sprouts, like bean and alfalfa, are totally acceptable. I also allow wheat grass, barley grass, and seaweed. Sauerkraut and kimchi are also acceptable, especially if they are organic and made from live cultures through a fermentation process.

I am not a fan of most soy products. Organic non-GMO soy protein and miso are the only soy products allowed on the REGENESIS program. There is a lot of argument and conflicting research concerning soy. DO NOT FEED SOY INFANT FORMULA PRODUCTS TO YOUR CHILDREN![4] Do not eat soy burgers or anything with soy oil, imitation meat products made from soy, soy milk, soy bars that have hydrolyzed soy proteins or any other kind of hydrolyzed proteins in them. Soy, a major endocrine disruptor, can cause thyroid dysfunction, heart disease, and cancer, especially estrogen driven cancers. Soy is one of the foods that is most often genetically modified. I have a lot of arguments over soy products, especially with steadfast vegetarians and others who think soy is the answer to world hunger. Read the book *The Whole Soy Story, The Dark Side of Americas Favorite Health Food,* by Dr. Kaayla Daniel.[5] This book is on my suggested reading list.

A great non soy based veggie burger is made by a company called Sunshine Burgers. They are gluten free, soy free, vegan, non-GMO verified, and contain quality organic ingredients. There are no "autolyzed" or "hydrolyzed" products in them. I highly recommend these burgers to my vegan and non-vegan friends and patients. If your health food store does not carry them, I feel certain they will order them for you. Their website is www.sunshineburger.com.

I get a lot of questions about protein shakes. I understand that it is easy to put a powder along with a fruit or some other ingredient in a blender and have a protein shake for breakfast. A lot of people are rushing around trying to get the kids off to school and get ready for work themselves. I get it. With proper planning and efficient time management, breakfast does not have to be a meal that is "skipped" because of time constraints. I recommend a healthy breakfast in the morning as it is one of the important goals of the REGENESIS program. If you must use a protein shake, make sure the soy based shakes are non-GMO and organic, the same goes for whey protein powders (I have a link to good protein powders at *regenesis4health.com*). Eating healthily and being healthy require some thought. Figure out how to have a wholesome breakfast every day.

Spices are OK on the program. It is best to buy them in bulk at the health food store. I prefer spices that are used in a lot of eastern type dishes like cumin, coriander, turmeric, cinnamon, nutmeg, curry, black and red pepper, chili, rosemary, parsley, and oregano. Spices make food taste great, provide variety, and have significant health value. Use them freely to taste.

Ketchup may be used if it is organic and free from high fructose corn syrup, but it should be used sparingly. The same holds true for mustard. Buy good quality organic mustard in small containers. Mayonnaise generally contains unhealthy oils and pasteurized eggs. I do not allow store bought mayonnaise to be used on the program. If you really want mayonnaise, find a recipe (you can find them online), and make a small amount of it. I have included a recipe for mayonnaise in the recipes chapter. Keep it in the fridge and throw it away after a couple of days.

Salt your food to taste! Don't go overboard here and use only sea salt. Quality sea salt is never white it's gray or pink in color. White iodized cheap table salt is not healthy, do not use it. Commercial salt is bleached and contains flow and non-caking agents. Sea salt is not cheap, but it is worth the extra money. Don't get me wrong here, salt like anything else can be done to excess. My second cousin was in the hospital following a "cardiac event" and the doctor put her on a salt restricted diet. I was visiting her and realized that she had been getting an IV of saline solution (salt water). Her blood tests revealed she was low in sodium, this always baffles me.

Quality and adequate salt is essential to life. If you have high blood pressure and eat a lot of commercially processed foods, you are probably getting too much "highly processed" salt. If you are dealing with hypertension or fluid retention issues, limit your exposure to salt and closely monitor your blood pressure, if elevated blood pressure persists, consult your doctor. Learn the salt content of your favorite foods and understand how much salt you are consuming every day. It is almost impossible to totally eliminate salt. Excess salts used in packaged foods are poor quality salts. If you are fully on the REGENESIS program and are not dealing with hypertension associated with fluid retention issues, use quality sea salt, and salt your food to taste.

I am sure that I left someone's favorite food out of my list. There are hundreds of foods available in America. There's no way I can mention them all. If you don't know about a certain food, just Google it. Do your own research and use your common sense. There is a wealth of information online. Include foods that you feel are within the guidelines of my program. Make sure to look at the carb content. A great website to research for food values is the USDA National Nutrient Database at http://www.nal.usda.gov/fnic/foodcomp/search/ .

Don't overeat! Eat slowly and chew your food. Use only a small glass of room temperature water when you eat. This prevents you from not chewing properly and then gulping your food down with a high volume of fluid. Eating slowly allows you to enjoy your food and keeps you from overeating. Don't eat late at night and then go to bed. This is a recipe for fatigue, insomnia and obesity.

It is worth learning the locations of local farmer's markets and stores that carry quality fresh organic foods in your area. Try to eat foods that are in season and fresh. Grow your own garden if you have the space to do so. Wash your fruits and vegetables thoroughly before eating them. Make cooking and preparing foods an important part of your daily routine. It is an art form and can be a lot of fun too. If cooking daily is a problem, prepare large portions and freeze the extra portions for those hectic days when there is no time to cook. Make soups and stews often as they are easily stored in freezer containers. "The Basic Soup" is okay to eat any time. It can be found in the recipe section that follows.

Learn about foods, how to cook quality delicious meals, how to plan ahead, and how and where to shop. It matters! Find some good cook books. One of my favorites is *The Primal Blueprint Cookbook*, by Mark Sisson.(6) Another favorite educational cook book on traditional foods is *Nourishing Traditions*, by Sally Fallon of the Westin A. Price Foundation (7) This book will also teach you about the history of various foods.

Phase 2

Phase 2 is added here to increase the food choices <u>after</u> you have reached health goals and are <u>fully in charge</u> of your appetite. I will allow beans like pinto's, Octobers, lima beans, adzuki beans, black beans, black eyed peas, etc. to be added to the food choices. Beans have a lot of nutritional value and contain beneficial fiber. Beans also contain fairly high amounts of carbohydrates, so you must be aware of this and factor it into your allowed daily carbohydrate intake. At this point it should be around 100 grams of carbs/day. A single bowl or a cup of beans would be acceptable a few times a week.

<u>If you are not a diabetic, and if you are not overweight</u>, you may add small servings of organic fruits back into your diet. Granny Smith apples, peaches, pears, and bananas (organic is preferred, as they have not been grown using toxic chemicals). If you live in areas where citrus fruits (oranges, and grapefruits) are grown, you may add small portions back into your diet. One of my food rules is <u>local grown</u> and in season. Bananas are my exception to this rule as they are not a citrus fruit and in many cases not locally grown (they are allowed). If possible, balance fruits with a protein like nuts, nut butters or cheese of some kind. Be careful about eating too much fruits and be aware of their carbohydrate content. Diabetics should avoid high sugar content fruits for the rest of their lives.

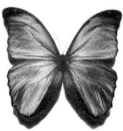

13

In Conclusion

"People are fed by the food industry which pays no attention to health, and are treated by the health industry that pays no attention to food."
Wendell Berry

WHERE DID THE REGENESIS PROGRAM COME FROM?

Over the years I have read countless diet books, South Beach Diet, Adkins Diet, The Mediterranean Diet, Primal Blueprint, The Zone Diet, The Jerusalem Diet, The pH Miracle, The Schwarzbein Principle, Eat Right 4 Your Type Diet, The Makers Diet, and countless others. I have learned a lot from all of them. I found things in all of them that I agree with and disagreed with. I have listened to many lectures by a lot of qualified individuals on diets, nutrition and supplementation. I have read thousands of pages of research and opinion articles in health journals and periodicals.

My nutritional instructor at Life University, Dr. Paul Goldberg, had a profound effect on my thinking very early on. In 2008, I met Dr. Joel Wallach in Chicago, his controversial message on mineral deficiencies and our love affair with wheat made a lot of sense to me. I attended several of the Weston A. Price Foundation meetings and listened to a plethora of wonderful speakers there. I received an incredible amount of information to chew on (pun intended). My good friend Robert Scott Bell introduced me to the massive influence of politics on health care. Add all of these influences together along with 14 years of clinical experience in dealing with real people with multiple health issues and that is where the diet portion of my program came from.

If we look at trends, they tell us a lot. The trend over the last 60+ years has been low fat, cholesterol restriction, and excess grain based carbohydrate consumption. We have seen an explosion of diseases and obesity. Can you see the result of our low fat, grain based food pyramid experiment? Just go to any shopping mall, a local street fair, Wal Mart, your local school, or the grocery store, and look at how unhealthy and overweight we Americans are. You do not have to be a researcher, scientist, or doctor to know this approach has failed and we must change course.

I have not spent time at a major research facility doing double blind placebo controlled studies. I have not measured twenty or thirty parameters related to body composition or blood values. Don't look for reviews of my work in any peer reviewed journal or on the evening news. What I am giving you is what works in my office for most people. It is not based on a complicated scientific model. It is merely based on some simple truths and empirical evidence that I have personally observed over the last 14 years and the hundreds of years of collective research I have read.

Most of the research we need to do regarding diet has already been done over and over again (millions of hours). I have read reams of it. We are talking about three major food groups here: fats, protein, and carbohydrates. They have been studied and mixed and analyzed a hundred different ways. Fad diets are just various combinations of these three components of food. It comes down to what we are willing to do, how much we understand our food choices, and to what length we are willing to go to protect and maintain our health. All I can do is offer my empirical advice based on my knowledge at this time. It is all rolled up in the REGENESIS program. I know that when patients follow the REGENESIS program guidelines, their abnormal blood values (sugars, A1C, and cholesterol) start to correct into the "normal" ranges. I see them lose weight and I watch many (sometimes all) of their health challenges decrease or resolve completely.

So when a patient asks me why I feel the way I do about suggesting free range meats, they might not understand that I have read hours upon hours of material on just that one thing and practiced it in my own life. I give them a ten second answer, a sound bite, as that is how we have been programed by radio and TV to receive information. There are very few people that are truly willing to dig down into the weeds for answers. So, they either trust my answer or they don't. Once they know that I have spent so much time on every little piece of my suggestions, they generally start to trust my advice. Know that every one of my recommendation has been thoroughly considered. I do not take the responsibility of these suggestions lightly. Some people think I'm crazy and will never take my advice. That's okay, we are free to believe what we choose.

What is continually changing is the way foods are produced and transported long distances in America. Our foods come from all over the world now. They are genetically modified, laced with preservatives, insecticides, growth hormones and who knows what else. Our world population is exploding. Scientists, universities and food industries all over the world are manipulating seeds and food manufacturing processes in order to feed this expansion. We are all going to pay the price in the long run with diseases, poor health, and shortened life-spans. It's already happening. It is very important to know what you are eating and to continually remain engaged in being healthy.

As you read the books that I have suggested, you will find some conflicting information and that's okay. Not everyone shares my philosophy exactly. I do not currently have a cookbook to offer (there may be one in the near future). As far as the cookbooks are concerned, try to find recipes that use foods allowed on the REGENESIS program. *The Primal Blueprint Cookbook* is one that is the closest to my dietary suggestions. Mr. Sisson and I share a very similar philosophy on foods.

Remember the foundational principals of my REGENESIS program are: Eliminate wheat, avoid all soft drinks, avoid processed sugars, and avoid all hydrogenated and rancid oils. Eat quality locally produced foods mostly non-starchy vegetables and drink pure water. Use quality supplementation appropriate for your body size. Reduce your exposures to environmental chemicals. These principals are crucial for your success. The other things we went over in this book are very important and will also add to your well-being and success.

We have covered a lot of things in the book. These things require understanding and then taking action. Keep in mind this is just the beginning. Continue to read and educate yourself regarding health. Make the necessary adjustments in your life. Set your goals! Understand the consequences of your actions. Own that you are largely responsible for your health situation. You must be the one to take control. Follow these guidelines, nourish your body properly and stay focused. Your good health destiny awaits you. Don't make excuses. You can do it! Recover your health! I want you to experience a REGENESIS!

Yours in health,
Dr. Garry Collins

REGENESIS Food List

This is a large list and there is plenty to choose from here.

- Eggs (free range)
- All meats (free range)
- Shrimp, lobster, crab, sea fish
- Fish (fresh water, not farm raised, no catfish)
- Salmon, deep sea fish (wild caught)
- Sweet Potatoes (organic is best)
- Lentils (1 small cup/day)
- All green leafy vegetables including:
    - Romaine lettuce
    - Green Leaf lettuce
    - Boston lettuce
    - Endive
    - Escarole
    - Spinach
    - Mustard greens
    - Collard greens
- Broccoli
- Cauliflower
- Brussels sprouts
- Leeks
- Dill pickles (organic)
- Asparagus
- Mushrooms
- Artichokes
- Avocados
- Squash (organic if possible)
- Zucchini (organic is best)
- Peppers (all kinds)
- Carrots
- Wild Rice (watch the carbs)
- Rice pasta (watch the carbs)
- Nuts (all kinds if no allergies)
- Almond milk (watch the carbs)
- Green beans
- Radishes
- Raw milk (in legal states)
- Quality cheese (not artificial)
- Lemon

Kale
Kohlrabi
Cabbage
Swiss Chard
Bok Choy
Cucumbers
Tomatoes
Celery

Garlic
Olives
Scallions
Onions
Pasta Sauce (organic only)
Steel Cut Oatmeal (1 small cup/day)
Nut Thins crackers ('watch the carbs')
Salsa (no sugars)

Lime
Blueberries
Blackberries
Raspberries
Strawberries (organic only)
Butter or ghee (organic)
Coconut oil (small container)
Olive oil (fresh in a small container)
All spices (fresh is preferred)
Sea salt (grey, brown or pink)
Ketchup (organic no HFCS)
Mustard (organic)
Stevia (drops only)
Almond/Cashew butter
Pomegranates (organic only)

REGENESIS Program Plan Summary

*Setting your goals short, medium, and long term.

*Drinking quality water and eliminating all man-made beverages.

*Eating wheat free.

*Avoiding sugars and harmful artificial sweeteners.

*Using butter and other quality fats, and eliminating rancid oils.

*Decreasing harmful poor quality Omega 6 fats and improving Omega 6:3 ratios

*Eating non-starchy carbohydrates, eggs and quality cuts of free range meats.

*Eliminating chemicals from your diet and your households.

*Taking quality supplementation appropriate to your body weight.

*Moving (exercising) properly for your current condition (do not move too quickly here).

*Considering and reducing your stress where you can.

*Thinking about the next book you need to read on your journey.

*Planning a vacation or at least something fun in the very near future.

*Following the eating guidelines.

*Staying focused and remembering how important your health is!

*Continuing to grow by seeking out information, reading all food labels, attending seminars, and knowing exactly what you are putting in your body. Challenge conventional thought.

*Passing your knowledge on to others with care and kindness because as you start to achieve results, there will be many who will ask you what you are doing. This will be true especially if you lose a lot of weight.

Recipes

These are a few starter recipes. You can find all kinds of recipes online and in other books.

Be creative!!

I have been using some of these recipes for years, I just make them and I can't remember where they came from. Any use without permission of someone's recipe is unintentional. Most of the recipes have undergone my personal twists and turns to get to where they are now.

Basic Soup

This is a variation of several recipes. The original idea for this soup came from Dianne Schwarzbein's "anytime soup", one of my patients brought me a cabbage soup recipe and I have included some of that recipe in "Basic Soup". Eat as much of this soup as you like. If you are hungry, it can be used as a meal or it can be used between meals. It is designed to get you through the tough times especially during the first part of the program. Be creative when making Basic Soup. Vary the ingredients as long as they are included in the allowable foods from the Eating Guidelines. The recipe below is just a basic starting point. Use different spices for variety.

6 to 8 cups of vegetable stock or water, you may also use meat broths. Read the ingredients on stock and broths! Many of them contain MSG, or hydrolyzed vegetable proteins.

3 to 4 chopped carrots
3 to 4 chopped celery stalks
1 to 2 diced tomatoes. (use to taste)
1 yellow squash and or zucchini (you can use either or both)
1 chopped onion
1 cup of shredded cabbage
1 cup of green beans (optional)
1 cup of frozen or fresh peas (optional)
1 or 2 cans of tomato sauce, or 1 or 2 small containers of V-8 juice (optional)

Salt to taste using real sea salt. Use any spices that you prefer
You may add more water or broth depending on how "thick" you prefer your soup
You do not have to use the tomato products if you don't like tomatoes
Place ingredients into a large soup pot and, cook for about 30 minutes over medium heat (gently boiling). Add more or less water or broth for desired consistency. Refrigerate and eat as much as you want. Throw away any leftover soup after 3 days. The Basic Soup can be frozen for future use.

GREEK SALAD
1 cup of finely chopped red or white onion (organic if possible)
1 teaspoon of vinegar or rice vinegar
1 teaspoon of fresh extra virgin olive oil
1 diced organic tomato
2 medium cucumbers finely sliced

Simply mix the ingredients in a medium to large bowl and serve
Serves 2

RED LENTIL SOUP
1 cup of red or green organic lentils
2 cups of organic vegetable or chicken broth
½ cup of chopped celery (organic if possible)
1 pound of free range chicken breasts chopped into small pieces
1 teaspoon of sea salt
½ cup of finely chopped organic onion
1 to 2 tablespoons of organic olive oil or butter
1 to 2 cloves of garlic (to taste)
1 teaspoon of parsley

Simmer lentils, chicken broth and chicken in a medium to large pot. Sautee onion garlic and celery in a frying pan using butter or olive oil, until onions are slightly brown. Combine the contents together in the large pot. Add parsley and salt. Simmer for 20 minutes.
Serves 4

SWEET POTATOES
2 medium organic sweet potatoes peeled and cut into 2 pieces
½ teaspoon of cinnamon powder (cinnamon verum is preferred)
4 pats of organic butter

Steam or boil the sweet potato cubes until soft. Place cooked sweet potatoes into 2 small bowls. Add a couple pats of butter to each bowl and drizzle with cinnamon powder.
Serves2

BUTTER SAUTED MUSHROOMS

2 cups of sliced mushrooms
2 tablespoons of organic butter
2 to 3 tablespoons of chicken or vegetable broth
Sea salt to taste
2 cloves of minced garlic or a small amount of diced onions, or both (your choice)
black pepper to taste

Sautee garlic and/or onion over medium heat in butter for 1 minute, add mushrooms and cook for 4 minutes. Add salt, pepper, and broth. Allow mixture to heat for 1 minute. Remove from heat.
Serves 2 or 3

EASY SPAGHETTI SQUASH PASTA

1 medium organic spaghetti squash cut in ½, remove the seeds
1 jar of your favorite pasta sauce (organic if possible)
½ lb. of free range hamburger (optional)

Place spaghetti squash in a large baking dish face down in ½ inch of water. Bake at 375 degrees for 30 minutes. Fry hamburger (optional). Remove squash from the oven, allow to cool for a few minutes. Heat your favorite spaghetti sauce. Combine spaghetti sauce with meat (optional). Remove spaghetti strings from squash length-wise into a medium bowl. Place desired spaghetti squash serving on a plate, add your favorite sauce, salt (with sea salt) and pepper to taste.
Serves 2 or 3

BAKED SALMON CAKES

1 can of Vital Choice wild caught canned salmon (they use BPA free cans!)
2 celery stalks finely chopped
½ cup of onion finely diced
2 teaspoons of parsley flakes
½ cup of organic coconut flour (optional)
1 medium or large free range egg

Preheat oven to 400 degrees. Clean salmon of bones and skin and put into a medium mixing bowl. Add onions, celery, parsley, coconut flour and egg. Mix with a fork until ingredients are completely combined. Pat out medium patties by hand and place on a cooking sheet (you can put a small amount of olive oil on the cooking sheet if desired to prevent sticking). Bake for 20 to 25 minutes or until brown. Remove and serve. If you like tomato sauce or ketchup on your cakes, use your favorite pasta sauce (heated) on top of the salmon cakes.
Serves 2

HEALTHY PIZZA

2 organic brown rice tortilla wraps
½ organic onion chopped
½ organic red, green, or yellow pepper chopped
1 small zucchini squash chopped
sliced olives (as many as you like)
Your favorite organic pasta sauce
1 to 2 cups of Mozzarella cheese
1 cup of free range hamburger or nitrite free bacon (free range nitrite free sausage is okay)

Preheat oven to 400 degrees. Place tortilla wraps on separate pizza sheets. Add sauce up to the edges. Place desired vegetable ingredients on

top of the sauce (use anything you want veggie wise) evenly distributed. Add hamburger or bacon (optional). Cover each pizza with cheese. Bake until cheese is melted (about 10 minutes). Allow to cool for a couple of minutes, slice and enjoy. If you are counting carbs (as you should) allow 30 grams of carbs for one tortilla wrap. (Remember 75 g of carbs per day is the sweet spot)
Serves 2 or 3

BAKED COD FISH
½ of a lemon (juice)
2 teaspoons of chopped rosemary
2 teaspoons of lemon pepper
1 tablespoon of extra virgin olive oil
4 codfish filets (5 to 7 oz. each)

Preheat oven to 350 degrees. Mix rosemary, lemon pepper, olive oil and lemon juice. Place washed fish fillets in a medium bowl and spread the mixture over each filet evenly. Bake on a cooking sheet or in a baking dish for 15 to 18 minutes.
Serves 4

MASHED CAULIFLOWER
1 head of organic cauliflower washed
Salt to taste
¼ to ½ cup of whipping cream
2 tablespoons of butter (optional)

Cut the stalk out of the cauliflower. You can cut the head of cauliflower into 5 or 6 pieces if you want. Boil until done, usually 10 to 15 minutes. Strain the cauliflower and put into a mixing bowl. Mix in butter and start to add whipping cream while blending with a blender on low speed

(a hand mixer will work too). Use enough whipping cream to get the desired texture. Salt to taste with sea salt.
Serves 2 or 3

GUACAMOLE
2 ripe avocados
½ lime (juice)
½ teaspoon sea salt
¼ cup of finely chopped onion (optional)

Peel and remove pit from avocados and place in a medium mixing bowl. Take a large fork and mash the avocado pieces until creamy. Add the lime juice, add salt, mix well. Add the onion (optional). Taste and add more lime and salt if desired. Goes well with salads, eggs in the morning, anything you can think of. Avocados are very healthy and a preferred food on the REGENESIS program.
Serves 2 or 3

POT ROAST
1 medium free range beef or bison chuck roast (3 to 4 lbs)
1 large onion (slice in half and then slice each half into quarters)
6 celery stalks sliced into 1 inch lengths
6 medium to large carrots sliced into 1 inch lengths
1 cup of water
1 bay leaf
1 tablespoon of sea salt
1 tablespoon of black pepper

Add water sea salt, pepper, bay leaf, and all of the other ingredients (except the roast) to the crock pot. Place the well washed chuck roast over top of the vegetables. Cover and cook for 4 ½ to 5 ½ hours on high setting or 9 to 10 hours on the low setting (covered). There are variations in crock pots so be sure to monitor your cooking times. Make adjustments accordingly. You may add sea salt and black pepper to taste after serving. Serves 5 to 7

EGGS

Eggs are a highly preferred food on the REGENESIS program. They should be free range farm raised eggs. There are many ways to prepare eggs. Poached is my favorite method or preparation followed by boiled and then lightly fried in organic butter. Eggs can be eaten over easy, poached or in omelet form with some of your favorite vegetables cooked into them.

Deviled eggs are a good way to eat eggs in the mornings if you don't have time to cook. They will store well for 3 or 4 days. Try using rice vinegar instead of mayonnaise when making deviled eggs. Celery, onion, celery seeds, mustard and pickles are ok to use. Pickles must not contain high fructose corn syrup (HFCS). This can be a challenging find as most pickles have HFCS in them. When boiling eggs, cover the eggs with about 1 inch of water. Bring them to a rolling boil and then remove them from the heat. Allow them to remain in the hot water for 15 to 20 minutes, pour off the warm water and fill pot with cold water.

Eggs have been falsley villified mainly because of their cholesterol content. Eating wheat, junk foods, soft drinks, food additives, sugar and stress are mostly what elevates cholesterol levels. Most people discover that very soon after starting the REGENESIS program that their cholesterol and triglyceride levels drop significantly. Do not believe the "food dictocrats" that say eggs are bad for you. Do not use egg substitutes. Eggs that pour out of a carton (box) are not natural or healthy. Buy free range eggs!

DEVILED EGGS AND PARMESAN

6 hard-boiled eggs
1 teaspoon of rice vinegar
2 teaspoon of lemon juice
¼ teaspoon of minced garlic
2 tablespoon. grated parmesan cheese

Slice hard boiled eggs into halves and hull out the yolks into a bowl. Blend all ingredients into the yolks except the parmesan cheese. Fill egg whites with mixture, sprinkle parmesan cheese over the egg halves.

SALADS

There are countless ways to make salads, just pick a base leaf lettuce that you prefer and add any of the vegetables that are allowed on the program. Use lemon or lime juice as dressing. Remember, if you are going to use olive oil on salads, I only allow olive oils that have been recently purchased in a small bottle and stored properly. Balsamic vinegar is also allowed. Try the juice of lemons or limes on salads, the taste will surprise you. Eat salads often and be creative in making them.

COLE SLAW

½ Head of shredded cabbage
1 small carrot shredded
3 tablespoons of rice vinegar
1 tablespoon of celery seeds

Combine cabbage and carrot and mix well. Add vinegar (use vinegar to taste) stir. Add celery seeds and stir. Ingredients can be adjusted according to your taste.
Serves 5 to 6

BAKED PORK CHOPS AND SWEET POTATOES
1 large onion cut into 8 wedges
¾ cup of MSG free chicken broth
2 tablespoons of Olive oil
2 large organic sweet potatoes peeled cut in half then into strips (about 20 strips)
1 teaspoon of fresh ginger (½ tsp. ginger powder can be substituted)
1 teaspoon of cinnamon
1 teaspoon of curry powder
4 thinly cut boneless pork chops

Preheat oven to 400 degrees. Coat large but shallow baking pan with olive oil. Place onions and sweet potatoes into pan. In a small bowl, add the seasonings, the oil and salt/pepper to taste. Drizzle this mixture over the onions and sweet potatoes. Roast in the oven and stir occasionally until the vegetables start to turn brown (about 30 minutes). Remove from oven, reduce oven temp to 375 degrees. Place pork chops over the onion and sweet potato mix, place in the oven for 15 minutes. Remove the pork chops and veggies into a bowl. Mix warmed chicken broth and any cooking juices from the baking pan together. Pour this mixture over the pork chops and veggies and serve. (26-28 g. carbs per serving, so add this into your daily carb calculation)
Serves 4

AMY'S BEEF STEW IN CLEAR BROTH
2 large sweet onions cubed
2 large sweet potatoes
1 cup of chopped mushrooms
1 bunch of parsley
3 cloves of garlic minced or sliced
2 lbs. of London Broil stew meat

2 tablespoons of sea salt
2 tablespoons of black pepper
1 cup of dry sherry

In a large crock pot, place onions on bottom, followed by sweet potatoes and then parsley. Place meat in next layer followed by mushrooms. Add salt, pepper and garlic. Cover ingredients with water. Cook on high for 2 hours. Add sherry. Cook on low heat for 8 hours. (Shared by my geek friend Amy Adams)
Serves 5 or 6

MAYONNAISE
1 egg yolk
2 tablespoons of lemon juice
¾ cup of extra virgin olive oil
1 tablespoon of dijon mustard (regular mustard will also work)

Use a food processor or a blender and blend lemon juice, mustard, and egg yolk until smooth. Slowly add oil until desired consistency is reached. Keep in the refrigerator for no more than 3 days.

Appendix

Suggested Reading

Note that there will be some information in these books that conflict with the information in the REGENESIS program. There has never been a book written in which I agree with everything the author writes. Some will say the same about my book. These are all good books on their own and I highly recommend them to my readers so that you may expand your knowledge of health. An asterisk means this book is very high on my reading list. Keep one in your reading rotation so that you may continue to educate yourself for the rest of your life. The knowledge you will acquire and the changes in your health will make you a magnet for people who are curious about how you recovered your health. Share your knowledge in a kind and thoughtful way.

The Sugar Blues by -William Dufty

Grain Brain – by Dr. David Perlmutter ***

The Great Cholesterol Con - by Anthony

Immortality - by Dr. Joel Wallach and Dr. Ma Lan ***

Death By Food Pyramid – by Denise Minger

Is This Your Child – by Doris Rapp MD

Toxic Beauty - by Dr. Samuel Epstein **

Detoxify Or Die – by Sherry Rodgers

The Power of Now - by Eckhardt Tolle

Your Erroneous Zone - by Dr. Wayne Dyer *

Primal Blueprint - by Mark Sisson **

The Primal Blueprint Cookbook – by Mark Sisson

The Schwarzbein Principle – by Dr. Diana Schwarzbein

Your Body's Many Cries for Water - by F. Batmanghelidj MD *

Wheat Belly - by Dr. William Davis***

Gut And Psychology Syndrome - by Dr. Natasha Campbell- McBride

The Omnivores Dilemma - by Michael Pollan

The Cholesterol Myths - by Uffe Ravnskov MD **

The Hidden Story of Cancer - by Brian Scott Peskin BSEE

The Politics of Cancer – by Dr. Samuel Epstein

Nutrition and Physical Degeneration - by Dr. Weston A. Price

Fast Food Nation - by Eric Schlosser

The Gut and Psychology Syndrome – by Natasha Campbell-McBride

'Excitotoxins' Tastes that Kill - by Dr. Russell Blaylock **

The Deadly Deception – by Mary Nash Stoddard

Splenda, Is It Safe or Not - by Dr. Janet Starr Hull

What's In This Stuff - by Patricia Thomas

The Safe Shoppers Bible - by Dr. Samuel Epstien *

Propaganda – by Edward Barnays

God Bless America – by Dr. Joel Wallach

Boundaries - by Henry Cloud and John Townsend *

Rare Earths, Forbidden Cures - by Dr. Joel Wallach

Who Will Cry When You Die - by Robin Sharma

Feelings Buried Alive - by Carol Truman

There is A Spiritual Solution To Every Problem – by Dr. Wayne Dyer

The Monk Who Sold His Ferrari – by Robin Sharma

Getting In the Gap – Wayne Dyer

The pH Miracle - by Dr. Robert O. Young

The Whole Soy Story, The Dark Side of America's Favorite Health Food - by Kaayla Daniel *

Nourishing Traditions – by Sally Fallon **

The Great Cholesterol Myth – by Dr. Stephen Sinatra and Johnny Bowden PhD. **

What Are You Hungry For- Depak Chopra MD. **

The Big Fat Surprise- Nin Teicholz. **

The Wahls Protocol- Dr. Terry Wahl MD. **

DVD's

The Oiling Of America – by Sally Fallon

Super Size Me – by Morgan Spurlock

Works Cited

Introduction
1. Perlmutter, David MD. *Grain Brain*. New York: Little, Brown and Company, 2013. P. 30 Print.
2. Ibid. P. 86
3. *How much money is spent on cancer research*. Nanomedicine center. com Web. accessed 1/14/14. <http://www.nanomedicinecenter.com/article/how-much-money-is-spent<
4. Heart Disease and Stroke Prevention. Centers for Disease Control and Prevention. Web. Accessed on 1/15/14. >http://www.cdc.gov/chronicdisease/rescources/publications/AAG/dhds<
5. USDA. *Profiling Food Consumption in America*. Web. Accessed 1/14/14. >www. usda. gov/factbook/chapter2.pdf<
6. Hyman, Mark MD. *Ultra Metabolism*. New York: Scribner, 2006. P. 60 Print.
7. Colpo, Anthony. *The Great Cholesterol Con*. United States: Self published, lulu.com. P. 60-74 Print.
8. Country Comparison." Life Expectancy At Birth." CIA (The World Factbook). Updated weekly. Web. Accessed 3/16/13. <http://www.cia.gov./library/publications/theworldfactbook/rankorder/2012rankhtml<

9. Infant Mortality (CIA World Factbook). Wikipedia. List of countries by infant mortality. Web. Accessed 1/14/14 >http://www.en.wikipedia.org/wiki/List_of_countries_by_infant_mort-ality_rate<

Chapter 1

1. Richards, Sir Mike. *"Extent and Cause of International Variations in Drug Use"* A report for the Secretary of State for health by Professor Sir Mike Richards CBE. Web. Accessed 3/16/13. >http://.dh.gov.uk/prod_consum_dh/groups/dh.digitalassets/@dh/@en/@ps/dc<
2. Carter, Jean. "Ill-Gotten Gains, The Rockefeller War on Drugs." Part 2,3,4. Rockefeller drugwars.com. N.d. Web. Accessed 3/29/12.
3. Rockwell, Llewellyn Jr. "Medical Control, Medical Corruption." N.d. http://www.Lewrockwell.com. (this article appeared in the June 1994 issue of Chronicles.) Web. Accessed 10/12/12.
4. Carter, James P. M.D. *Racketeering In Medicine*. Virginia: Hampton Roads Publishing Company Inc.1993. P. xxvii Print.
5. Duffy, Thomas P. M.D. "The Flexner Report – 100 Years Later." *Yale Journal of Biology and Medicine*. 2011 September, 84(3): 269-276 Web. Accessed 10/4/13.
6. Richardson, Martyn E. "Tracing The Decline of OMT in Patient Care." *Journal of The American Osteopathic Association* July, 2006. Vol. 106 No. 7, P. 378-379.
7. Starfield, Barbara –MD MPH. " Is US Health Really the Best in the World?" *JAMA,* 26 July 2000. Vol. 284, No. 4, P. 483.
8. Ibid.
9. Dr. Joel Wallach (in many of his public lectures has said this hundreds of times).
10 Life Expectancy at Birth. CIA- The World Factbook. Web. Accessed 1/14/14. >https://www.cia.gov/library/publications/the-world-factbook/rankorde<

11. Country Comparison. "Life Expectancy At Birth." CIA (the World Factbook). Updated weekly. Web. Accessed 3/16/13. <http://www.cia.gov./library/publications/theworldfactbook/-rankorder/2012rankhtml<

12. Stoxen, Colleen. "Only 8% from pink NFL merch. goes to breast cancer research." Star Tribune/Lifestyle. 16 Oct. 2013. Web Accessed 10/28/13. >http://www.startribune.com/lifestyle/blogs/228073131.html<

13. Wallach, Joel, Ma Lan MD. *Immortality*. CA: Wellness Publications LLC, 2008. P. 39 Print.

14. Ibid. P. 136-138

15. Kushi, Michio, Stephen Blauer. *The Macrobiotic Way (3rd edition)*. New York: Avery (Penguin Group), 2004. E-book, Chapter 5 (no page listed).

16. Minger, Denise. *Death by Food Pyramid*. CA: Primal Blueprint Publishing, 2013. Print.

17. Enig, Mary, PhD, Sally Fallon. *"The Oiling of America"*. Originally printed in Nexus Magazine in 2 parts, Nov/Dec 98 and Feb/Mar99. Web Accessed 3/17/2013. <http://www.drcranton.com/nutrition/oiling.htm<

18. Wallach, Joel ND, Ma Lan MD. *God Bless America*. CA: Wellness Publications LLC, 2013. P. 16 Print.

19. Sears, Barry PhD. *Enter The Zone*. New York: Harper Collins Publishing, Inc., 1995 Print.

20. Wallach, Joel, Ma Lan MD. *Rare Earths Forbidden Cures*. CA: Double Happiness Publishing Co., 1996. P. 141 Print.

21. Epstein, Samuel MD, Randall Fitzgerald. *Toxic Beauty*. Texas: Ben Bella, Inc., 2009. P. 2 Print.

22. "Overmedication in Seniors" No author. *Resources for Seniors Inc.*, 27 Feb. 2007. Web Accessed 10/29/13. >www.resourcesforseniors.com/pharm_essays/overmedication.doc<

Chapter 2

1. Perlmutter, David MD. *Grain Brain*. New York: Little, Brown and Company 2013. P. 181-182 Print.
2. Batmanghelidj, F. MD. *Your Body's Many Cries For Water*. Virginia: Global Health Solutions Inc., 1995. Print.
3. Ibid P. 5
4. Marks, Jay W. MD. *Constipation*. MedicineNet.com. 19 Aug. 2012. Web. Accessed 3/17/13. <http://www.medicinenet.com/constipation/page2.htm<
5. Wallach, Joel, Ma Lan MD. *Immortality*. CA: Wellness Publications LLC, 2008. P. 267 Print.
6. Williams, David. *The Acid Reflux/Soda Connection*. Dr. David Williams website. 23 Aug. 2012. Access 17 Mar. 2013. Web. <http://www.drdavidwilliams.com/acid-reflux-and-soda-connection#ax222NqPRY6<
7. Wallach, Joel ND, Ma Lan MD. *God Bless America*. CA: Wellness Publications LLC, 2013. P. 71-72 Print.
8. Berkow, Robert MD, Andrew Fletcher, et al. *The Merk Manual*. NJ: Merck Research Laboratories, 1992. P. 1356-1357 Print.
9. Wallach, Joel, Ma Lan MD. *Immortality*. CA: Wellness Publications LLC, 2008. P. 267 Print.
10. Wallach, Joel ND. Ma Lan MD. *God Bless America*. CA: Wellness Publications LLC, 2013. P. 199 Print.
11. Browner, Carol (Administrator of the US EPA under the Clinton administration). "Pesticides in Drinking Water." 18 Oct. 1994. Web Accessed 10/8/2013. >http://psep.cce.cornell.edu/issues/pesticides-water.aspx<
12. Garcia, Gregory Bren. "Guide to Plastic Safety: WhatYou Need to Know About Plastic Resin Codes." Smart Parenting.com. 3 Sept. 2010. Web. Accessed 11/2/13. >http://www. smartparenting.com.ph/homeliving/homebase/guide-to-plstic-safety-what-you-need-to-know-about-plastic-resin-codes<

13. Ibid.
14. Browner, Carol (Administrator of the US EPA under the Clinton administration). "Pesticides in Drinking Water." 18, Oct. 1994. Web Accessed 10/18/2013. >http://psep.cce.cornell.edu/issues/pesticides-water.aspx<

Chapter 3
1. Davis, William MD. *Wheat Belly.* New York: Rodale, 2011. P. 26-27 Print.
2. Ibid. P.21
3. Allbritton, Jen, CN. "Wheaty Indiscretions: What Happens to Wheat, from Seed to Storage." Weston A. Price Foundation. 30 June 2003. Web. Accessed 10/10/13. >http://www. westonaprice.org/modern-foods/wheaty-indiscretions<
4. Sardi, Bill. "Just How Many Americans Did Vioxx Kill?" LewRockwell.com. 21 April, 2006. Web, Accessed 10 Oct. 2013.>http://www.lewrockwell.com/2006/04/bill-sardi/just-how-many-americans-did-vioxx-kill/<
5. Senate Document #264. Better Health Thru Research. Web Accessed 9/26/13. >http://betterhealththruresearch.com/document264htm.<
6. Allbritton, Jen, CN. "Wheaty Indiscretions: What Happens to Wheat, from Seed to Storage." Weston A. Price Foundation. 30, June 2003. Web. Access 10 Oct. 2013. >http://www. -westonaprice.org/modern-foods/wheaty-indiscretions<
7. Perlmutter, David MD. *Grain Brain.* New York: Little, Brown and Company, 2013. P. 23-67 Print.
8. Davis, William MD. *Wheat Belly.* New York: Rodale, 2011. P. 9-10 Print.
9. Ibid P. 33-34.
10. Hyman, Mark MD. "Why Cholesterol May Not Be the Cause Of Heart Disease." Huffington Post, June 28, 2012. >http://www.huffingtonpost.com/dr-mark-hyman/why-cholesterol-may<

11. Lipinski, Elizabeth. *Leaky Gut Syndrome*. Los Angeles: Keats Publishing, 1998. P. 9-17 Print.
12. Ibid. P. 9
13. Reproducibility and Viability of ALCAT Testing. Web Accessed 12/9/13. >https://www.alcat.com/pages/reproducibility-viability/<
14. Sherman, Carl. "Early recognition of atypical celiac disease." The Clinical Advisor. April 2009. Web. Accessed 3/26/14. >http://www.clinicaladvisor.com/early-recognition-of-atypical-celiac-d..<
15. Davis, William MD. *Wheat Belly*. New York: Rodale, 2011. P. 58-94 Print.
16. Kaseem, Noreen. "Baby Wheat Allergy Symptoms." Livestrong.com. 23 May 2012. Web. Accessed 10/10/13. >*http://www.livestrong.com/article/129876-baby-wheat-allergy-symptoms/*<
17. Hadjivassiliou M, Kandler RH, Chattopadhyay AK, et al. "Dietary treatments of gluten neuropathy." *Muscle Nerve* 2006 Dec; 34(6):762-6.
18. Hafstrom I, Ringertz B, Spangberg A, et al. "A vegan diet free of gluten improves the signs and symptoms of rheumatoid arthritis: the effects on arthritis correlate with a reduction in antibodies to food antigens." *Rheumatoid* 2001; 1175-9.
19. West J, Logan R, Smith C, et al. "Malignancy and mortality in people with celiac disease: population based cohort study." *Brit Med J* 2004 July21;doi:10.1136/bmj.38169.486701.7C.
20. Perlmutter, David MD. *Grain Brain*. New York: Little, Brown and Company, 2013. P. 84-86 Print.
21. McBride, Natasha MD. *Gut and Psychology Syndrome*. United Kingdom: Medinform Publishing. 5th reprint 2011. Print.
22. Perlmutter, David MD. *Grain Brain*. New York: Little, Brown and Company, 2013. P. 149-177 Print.
23. Ibid.
24. Smith, Jeffrey. "Are Genetically Modified Foods a Gut-Wrenching Combination?" Institute for Responsible Technology. Nov. 2013.

Web. Accessed 2/1/2014. >http://responsibletec- hnology.org/glutenintroduction<
25. Allbritton, Jen CN. "Wheaty Indiscretions: What Happens to Wheat, from Seed to Storage." Weston A. Price Foundation. 30 June 2003. Web. Accessed 10/10/13. >http://www. westonaprice.org/modern-foods/wheaty-indiscretions<
26. Davis, William M.D. *Wheat Belly*. New York: Rodale, 2011. P. 12-30 Print.

Chapter 4

1. Bowden, Johnny Ph.D, Sinatra, Stephen MD. *The Great Cholesterol Myth*. E-book P.
2. Dufty, Patrick. *The Sugar Blues*. New York: Warner Books Inc., 1975 (re-issue 1993). Print. Original printing- PA: Clarence Williams Publishing Co., 1949; PN: Chilton Book Company, 1975. P. 13-27 Print.
3. Ibid. P.110-115
4. Pollan, Michael. *The Omnivores Dilemma*. New York: The Penguin Press, 2006. Print.
5. Methylphenidate, or Ritalin, is Very Similar to Cocaine/Crack. Neuro Soup. June 3, 2014. Web. Accessed 6/3/2014. >http://www.neurosoup.com/ritalin-is-similar-to/<
6. McBride, Natasha MD. *Gut and Psychology Syndrome*. United Kingdom: Medinform Publishing. 5th reprint 2011. P. 117-219. Print
7. Rapp, Doris MD. *Is This Your Child?* New York: William Morrison and Company Inc., 1991. Print
8. Irwin, Kim. "Pancreatic cancers use fructose, common in Western diet, to fuel growth, study finds." UCLA Newsroom. 1 Feb. 2014. Newsroom. Web. Accessed 2/1/2014. >http://newsroom.ucla.edu/portal/ucla/panxreatic-pancreatic-cancers-use-fructose<
9. Ibid.

10. Peskin, Scott. *The Hidden Story of Cancer.* Texas: Pinnacle Press, 2006. P.148 Print.
11. Ibid. p.
12. Positron Emission Tomography. Wikipedia. Web. Accessed 2/1/2014.
13. Dufty, Patrick. *The Sugar Blues.* New York: Warner Books Inc., 1975 (re-issue 1993). Print. Original printing- PA: Clarence Williams Publishing Co., 1949; PN: Chilton Book Company, 1975. Print.
14. The Glycemic Index, Wikipedia. Web. Accessed 1/25/2014.
15. Schwarzbein, Diana MD, Nancy Deville. *The Schwarzbein Principle.* Florida: Health Communications Inc., 1999 Print.
16. Schwarzbein, Diana MD, Nancy Deville, Evelyn Jacob Jaffee. *The Schwarzbein Principle Vegetarian Cookbook.* FL: Health Communications Inc.,1999. P, 2 Print.

Chapter 5

1. Wallach, Joel ND Ma Lan MD. *God Bless America.* CA: Wellness Publications LLC, 2013. P. 90 Print.
2. Schmid, Ron ND. "Food Supplements, Weston A. Price & Nutritional Principles." 2008, Web. Accessed 10/2/13.
3. Crisco (history). "Crisco Is Introduced". www.Crisco.com. Web. Accessed 10/3/13.
4. Schmid, Ron ND. "Food Supplements, Weston A. Price & Nutritional Principles." 2008.Web. Accessed 10/2/13
5. Weston A. Price Foundation. Wikipedia. Web. Accessed 10/3/13.
6. Price, Weston A. *Nutrition and Physical Degeneration.* New York. Medical Book Dept. of Harper & Brothers. Paul B. Hoeber, Inc. 1939. Print.
7. Fallon, Sally. "Dirty Little Secrets of the Food Processing Industry." Weston A. Price Foundation. 26 Dec. 2005. Web. Accessed 4/28/12. >http://www.westonaprice.org/modernfoods / dirty-secrets-of-the-food-processing-ind<

8. Shlosser, Eric. *Fast Food Nation*. New York: Houghton Mifflin Co. 2001
9. Spurlock, Morgan. Super Size Me. The Con Production Co. 2004.
10. O'Brien, Richard. *Fats and Oils: Formulating and Processing for Applications*. New York: CRC Press LLC, 2004. P. 59
11. Ibid. P. 59
12. Ibid. P. 13
13. Davis, William MD. *Wheat Belly*. New York: Rodale, 2011. P. 28-29 Print.
14. Weil, Andrew MD. "Is Cottonseed Oil Okay?" Q& A Library. www.Drweil.com. Web. Accessed 10/3/13.
15. Wallach, Joel, Ma Lan MD. *Immortality*. CA: Wellness Publications LLC, 2008. P. 51 Print.
16. Senate Document #264. Better Health Thru Research. Web. Accessed 9/26/13. >http://betterhealththruresearch.com/document264htm<.
17. Curzons, Farley. "Thought For Food." The East Shore Mainstreet. Year 21, Number 6, June 2011. Web. Accessed 2/6/14. >mainstreet.eshore.ca/back_issue/2011/June_2011_Main_street.pdf<
18. Enig, Mary PhD, Fallon Sally. *"The Oiling of America."* Dr. Cranton.com. Web. Accessed 2/17/12. >http://drcranton.com/nutrition/oiling.htm<. Side note: this was originally published in Nexus Magazine in 2 parts, Nov/Dec 1998 and Feb/Mar 1999 and was published by Dr. Cranton with permission from the authors. It is available online at the address above.
19. Ravnskov, Uffe MD. *The Cholesterol Myths*. Washington DC: New Trends Publishing Inc. 2000. P.9-95
20. Chowdhury, Rajiv MD. PhD, et al. "Association of Dietary, Circulating, and Supplement Fatty Acids With Coronary Risk: A Systematic Review and Meta- Analysis." *Annals of Internal Medicine*. 18 March 2014; Vol 160(6):398-406.
21. Hyman, Mark MD. "Why Cholesterol May Not Be the Cause Of Heart Disease." Huffington Post, 28 June 2012.>http://www.

huffingtonpost.com/dr-mark-hyman/why-cholesterol-may<.

22. Wallach, Joel, Ma Lan MD *Immortality.* CA: Wellness Publications LLC, 2008. P. 3 Print.
23. "Principles of Healthy Diets." Weston A Price Foundation. 1 Jan. 2000. Web. Accessed 4/28/12. P. 9. No specific author given. >http://www.westonaprice.org/basics/prin- ciples-of-healthy-diets<
24. Ibid.
25. Teichloz, Nina. *The Big Fat Lie.* New York: Simon & Schuster 2014. Print.
26. Siri, Tarino. "Saturated fat, carbohydrate, and cardiovascular disease." *The American Journal of Cllinical Nutrition.* 20 Jan. 2010. March 2010 Vol. 91 No. 3 P. 502-509.
27. Colpo, Anthony. *The Great Cholesterol Con.* United States: Self published, lulu.com. P. 60-74 Print.
28. Enig, Mary PhD, Fallon Sally. *"The Oiling of America."* Dr. Cranton.com. Web. Accessed 2/17/12 >http://drcranton.com/nutrition/oiling.htm. Side note: this was originally published in Nexus Magazine in 2 parts, Nov/Dec 1998 and Feb/Mar 1999 and was published by Dr. Cranton with permission from the authors. It is available online at the address above.
29. Lundberg GD, Voigt GE, "Reliability of a presumptive diagnosis in sudden unexpected deaths in adults." *Journal of the American Medical Association* 242, 2328-2330. 1979
30. Kirchner T, et al. "The autopsy as a measure or accuracy of the death certificate." *New England Journal of Medicine* 1985 Nov 14;313(20)1263-1269.
31. Ravnskov, Uffe MD. *The Cholesterol Myths.* Washington DC: New Trends Publishing Inc. 2000. P.9-95
32. Bowden, Johnny PhD, Sinatra, Stephen MD. *The Great Cholesterol Myth.*
33. Enig, Mary PhD, Fallon Sally. *"The Oiling of America."* Dr. Cranton.

com. Web. Accessed 2/17/12. >http://drcranton.com/nutrition/oiling.htm.< Side note: this was originally published in Nexus Magazine in 2 parts, Nov/Dec 1998 and Feb/Mar 1999 and was published by Dr. Cranton with permission from the authors. It is available online at the address above.
34. Null, Gary, PhD, Jerry Stillman. "Medicine for Sale: Tracing the Shadowy Money Trail that Exploits your Health (Part1)" Gary Null blog. Dec/12/2011. Web. Acceessed 3/17/14. >gnasquarespace.com/home/medicine-for-sale-tracing-the-shadowy-money-trail-that-explo.html<
35. Matsuzaki M, et al. "Large Scale Cohort Study of the relationship between serum cholesterol concentration and coronary events with low dose simvistatin therapy in Japanese patients with hypercholest erolemia."*Circulation Journal.* Dec. 2002; 66 (12):1087-1095.
36. Zueric M, et al. "Decline in serum total cholesterol and the risk of death from cancer." *Epidemiology.* Mar. 1997; 8 (2):137-143.
37. Ellison LF, Morrison HI. "Low serum cholesterol concentration and risk of suicide." *Epidemiology,* Mar. 2001; 12 (2): 168-172.
38. Waters, David, Jenifer E. Ho, David A. Demicco, et al. "Predictors of New-Onset Diabetes in Patients Treated With Atorvastin." *JACC (Journal of American Cardiology).* April 2011, Issue 14.
39. Culver, Annie L, et al. "Statin Use and Risk of Diabetes Mellitus in Postmenopausal Women in the Women's Health Initiative." *Archives of Internal Medicine* 2012, 172(2):144-152. Web. Accessed 10/3/13
40. Clodagh S.M. O'Gorman, Michael B. O'Neil, Louise S. Conwell. "Considering statins for cholesterol-reduction in children if lifestyle and diet changes do not improve their health: a review of the risks and benefits." *Vascular Health Risk Management.* 2011; 7:1-14, published online 2010 December 20. Web Accessed 10/2/13. >http://www.lenus.ie/hse/handle/1047/135096<
41. Marchione, Marilynn. "US Doctors urge wider use of cholesterol

drugs" Assoc. Press. 13 Nov. 2013. Web. Accessed 2/4/2014. >http://news.yahoo.com/us-doctors-urge-wider-chol-esterol-drugs-213<

42. Heart Disease and Stroke Prevention. *Centers for Disease Control and Prevention*. Web. Accessed on 1/15/14. >http://www.cdc.gov/chronicdisease/rescources/publications/AAG/dhds<

43. Virgin, JJ. CNS, CHFS. *The Virgin Diet*. Ontario: Harlequin. 2012. P 21, 127-128.

44. Destination Heart Healthy Eating. Bell Institute of Health and Nutrition. 2009 General Mills. HH 300, (A pamphlet) no author's name given.

45. Frank B. Hu, et al. "Meta-analysis of Prospective Cohort Studies Evaluating The Association of Saturated Fat with Cardiovascular Disease" *American Journal of Clinical Nutrition* 91, no.3(2010):502-9.

46. A.W. Weverling-Rijnsburger, et al., "Total Cholesterol and Risk of Mortality in the Oldest Old," *Lancet* 350, no9085 (October 18, 1997): 1119-23.

47. Rizvi, Kash, John P. Hampson, John N. Harvey. "Do lipid-lowering drugs cause erectile dysfuncrtion? A systematic review." *Family Practice* (2002) 19 (1): 95-98. Web. Accessed 11/25/2013. >http://fampra.oxfordjournals.org/content/19/1/95.short<

48. Perlmutter, David MD. *Grain Brain*. New York: Little Brown and Co. 2013. P. 30

49. Seneff, Stephanie. "APOE-4: the Clue to Why Low Fat Diet and Statins may Cause Alzheimer's." 4/26/11 Web. Accessed 11/25/2013. >http://people.csail.mit.edu/seneff/alzheimer's_statins.html<

50. Nordestguaard, BG, Benn M, Schnohr P, et al. "Non-fasting triglycerides and risk of myocardial infarction, ischemic heart disease, and death in men and women." *JAMA 2007* Jul 18;298(3):299-308

51. Johnson, Jo. "Health Benefits of Grass Farming" Rain Crow Ranch/American Grass Fed Beef. Web. Accessed on 11/27/2013. >http://www.americangrassfedbeef.com/grass-fed-natural-beef.asp<

52. Davis, William MD. *Wheat Belly.* New York: Rodale, 2011. P. 146-153 Print.
53. Siri-Tarino. "Saturated fat, carbohydrate, and cardiovascular disease." *The American Journal of Clinical Nutrition.* 20 Jan. 2010. March 2010 vol.91 no. 3 502-509.
54. Bowden, Johnny PhD, Sinatra, Stephen MD. *The Great Cholesterol Myth.* E-book P. 255.

Chapter 6
1. Blaylock, Russel MD. *Excitotoxins- The TasteThat Kills,* NM:Health Press, 1997. P. xxi, 107, 168-169 Print.
2. Ibid. P. xix, xxi Print.
3. Ibid. P. 34
4. Olney, J.W. "Excitotoxic Food Additives: Functional Teratological Aspects." *Prog. Brain Res.* 18(1998):283-294.
5. Mercola, Joseph MD. "FDA Slammed for Calling BPA Safe." 20 Nov. 2008. Mercola.com. Web. Accessed 5/13/2012. >http://articles.mercola.com/sites/articles/archive/2008/ 11/20/fda-slammed<
6. Ibid.
7. Scanlan, Richard A, "Nitrosamines and Cancer." The Linus Pauling Institute. Nov. 2000. Web. Accessed 2/1/2014. >http://lpi.oregonstate.edu/f-w00/nitrosamine.html<
8. Mercola, Joseph MD. "The Psychosis-Inducing Beverage Ingredient You've probably Never Heard Of." 11 Jan. 2012. Mercola.com. Web. Accessed 5/13/12. >http://articles.mercola. com/sites/articles/archive/2012/01/11/brominated<
9. Ibid. From the above article subcaption- "Health Risks of Bromine" from an audio interview with physician Jorge Flechas.
10. PepsiCo replacing Gatorade ingredient after online petition. Reuters 25 Jan. 2013. Web. Accessed 11/9/13. > http://www.reuters.com/assets/print?aid=USBRE9O017D20130125<

11. Aspartame, Wikipedia. Web. Accessed on 2/21/2012. >http://wikipedia.org/wiki/ aspatame<
12. Blaylock, Russel MD. *Excitotoxins: Taste That Kills,* NM:Health Press, 1997. Print. P. 68-70
13. Tivana, Michael "Nutra-Sweet" Tribal Messenger. 12 Mar. 1991 and a 2004 update. Web. Accessed 6/10/12. >http://www.tribalmessenger.org/columns/nutrasweet.htm<
14. Stoddard, Mary Nash. *The Deadly Deception.* Texas: Odenwald Press. 1998. Print
15. Smith, Lendon MD. "Greed vs. Health, Which Will Win?" Aspartame Consumer Safety Network Fact Sheet. Web. Accessed 6/10/12. >http://healthread.net/aspfactshtm
16. Corsi, Hector E. "Study: Aspartame linked to blood cancers." Digital Journal, 7 Nov. 2012. Web. Accessed 11/11/12. >http://digitaljournal.com/article/336384
17. Mercola, Joseph MD. "New Study of Splenda Reveals Shocking Information About Potential Harmful Effects." Mercola.com. Web. Accessed 5/13/12.>http://articles.mercola.com/sites/articles/archive/2009/02/New-study
18. Ibid.
19. Hull, Janet Starr MD, Lynn Dealey. *Splenda, Is It Safe Or Not.* Texas: The Pickle Press, 2004. Print.
20. Shenker, Maura. "Side Effects of Using Agave Syrup." Livestrong.com. Web.Accessed 12/12/13. >http://livestrong.com/article/308147-side-effects-of-using-agave-syrup/<
21. "Toxicity from gum, Candy, and Toothpaste in Dogs." Pet MD. Web. Accessed 2/14/ 2014. >http://www.petmd.com/dog/conditions/endocrine/c_dg_xylitol_toxicity<
22. "Sample quotes from cancer expert's letters on acesulfame testing." CSPI, Web. Accessed 5/20/1212. >http://www.cspnet.org/reports/asekquot.html<

23. The Delaney Clause. Wikipedia. Web. Accessed 12/10/12.
24. Scott vs. FDA. *The Delaney Clause Challenged.* United States Court of Appeals, Sixth Circuit. Argued Jan 25, 1984, Decided Feb 23, 1984. Web. Accessed 10/12/13. >http://openjurist. org/728/f2d/322/mw-scott-v-food-and-drug-administration<
25. Acrylamide. Wikipedia. Web. Accessed 10/10/2013.
26. Kobylewski, Sarah, Michael F. Jacobsen PhD. "Food Dyes A Rainbow of Risks." Center for Science in the Public Interest. 2010. Web. Accessed 10/10/2013. >http://cspinet.org/new/pdf/food-dyes-rainbow-of-risks.pdf
27. Dr. Benjamin Feingold. Wikipedia. Web. Accessed 12/6/13. >http://en.wikipedia.org/wiki/Benjamin-Feingold
28. Hattis, D., R. Goble, et al. "Age Related Differences in Susceptibility to Carcinogenesis: A Quantitative Analysis of Empirical Animal Bioassay Data." *Environmental Health Perspectives.* 2005,113:509-516.
29. Kobylewski, Sarah, Michael F. Jacobsen PhD. "Food Dyes A Rainbow of Risks." Center for Science in the Public Interest. 2010. Web. Accessed 10/10/13.. >http://cspinet.org/new/pdf/ food-dyes-rainbow-of-risks.pdf<
30. "But aren't the FD&C dyes certified to be safe?" Untitled from Feingold.org. Web. Accessed 2/17/2014. >http://feingold.org/certified.php<
31. Scott vs. FDA. *The Delaney Clause Challenged.* United States Court of Appeals, Sixth Circuit. Argued Jan 25, 1984, Decided Feb 23, 1984. Web. Accessed 12 Oct. 2013. >http:// openjurist.org/728/f2d/322/mw-scott-v-food-and-drug-administration<
32. Kobylewski, Sarah, Michael F. Jacobsen PhD. "Food Dyes A Rainbow of Risks." Center for Science in the Public Interest. 2010. Web. Accessed 10/10/13.. >http://cspinet.org/new/pdf/ food-dyes-rainbow-of-risks.pdf<

Chapter 7

1. Worldwatch Institute. "POP's Culture." Jan.2, 2014. Web. Accessed 1/2/14. >http://www.worldwatch.org/noce485<
2. Are Pharmaceuticals present in the environment? Department of Ecology State of Washington. Web. Accessed 1/6/14. >http://www.ecy.wa.gov/programs/htwr/pharmaceuticals/ pages/pie.html<
3. Browner, Carol. "Pesticides in Drinking Water." Cornell University Cooperative Extension. Oct. 18, 1994. Web. Accessed 10/8/2013. >http://psep.cce.cornell.edu/issues/pesticides-water.aspx<
4. Wikipedia. "Jacqueline Kennedy Onasis." Web. Accessed Jan 9, 2014. >Wikipedia. org/wiki/Jacqueline_Kennedy_Onasis.<
5. Peter Lamas.com. Web. Accessed 1/2/2014. >www.PeterLamas.com/cophilosophy.php<
6. Epstein, Samuel MD. Randall Fitzgerald. *Toxic Beauty*. Texas: Ben Bella, Inc., 2009. Print.
7. Epstein, Samuel M.D. *The Politics of Cancer.* New York: East Ridge Press, 1998. Print.
8. Morgan, Graeme, Robyn Ward, Michael Barton. "The Contribution of Cytotoxic Chemotherapy to 5-Year Survival in Adult Malignancies." Clinical Oncology (2004) 16:549-560
9. Ubel, Peter MD. "Who Pays Your Oncologist?" *Psychology Today*. Published on May 30, 2012 in Critical Descisions. Web. Accessed 1/6/2014. >http://www.psychologytoday.com/blog/critical-descisions/201205/who-pays-your-oncologist<
10. Mercola, Joseph MD. "Are You Poisoning Your Household With this Chore?" Mercola.com. Dec. 2011. Web. Accessed 12/25/2011. >http://aarticles.mercola.com/sites/ articles/archive/2011/12/21/are-you<
11. Priesnitz, Wendy. "Air Fresheners or Air Pollutants?" *Natural Life Magazine*. Web. Accessed 1/14/14. >http://www.naturallifemagazine.com/0810/airfresheners.htm<

12. Rogers, Sherry A. MD. *Detoxify or Die*. Florida, Sand Key Company Inc., 2002. P. 10-18 Print.
13. Faber, Scott. Neka, Leiba. "Exposing The Cosmetics Cover-Up." Environmental Working Group. Web. Accessed on 1/8/2014. >http://www.ewg.org/research/exposing-cosmetics-cover/toxic-chemicals<
14. Epstein, Samuel M.D., Randall Fitzgerald. *Toxic Beauty*. Texas: Ben Bella, Inc. 2009. P, 157-159 Print.
15. "Pollution Prevention and Toxics." United States Environmental Protection Agency (7407). OPPT Chemical Fact Sheet. Feb. 1995. Web. Accessed 2/12/2014. >http://www.epa.gov/ chemicalfact/dioxa-sd.txt<
16. Epstein, Samuel M.D., Randall Fitzgerald. *Toxic Beauty*. Texas: Ben Bella, Inc. 2009. P, 19 Print.
17. Dabre PD., et al. "Concentrations of Parabens in Human Breast Tumors."*Journal of Applied Toxicology*. (2004) Jan-feb;24(1):5-13
18. Genius, Stephen J. "Nowhere to hide: Chemical toxicants and the unborn child." *Reproductive Toxicology*. 28 (2009) 115-116
19. "Bisphenol A." U.S. Food & Drug Administration. FDA.gov. Food Ingredients Packaging. Web.Accessed 3 Jul. 2012.>http://www.fda.gov/FoodIngredientsPackaging/ucm166145.htm<
20. Rogers, Sherry MD. *Detoxify or Die*. Florida:Sand Key Company Inc. 2002. Print.
21. Thomas, Patricia. *What's In This Stuff*. New York: 2008. Penguin Group (USA) Inc. Print.
22. Epstein, Samuel MD., Fitzgerald, Randall. *Toxic Beauty*. Texas: Ben Bella, Inc. 2009. Print. P, 68
23. Epstein, Samuel MD. *The Politics of Cancer.* New York: East Ridge Press, 1998. Print. P.569
24. Epstein, Samuel MD., Randall Fitzgerald. *Toxic Beauty*. Texas: Ben Bella, Inc. 2009. Print. P. 52

25. Ibid. P. 54
26. Epstein, Samuel MD., *The Safe Shoppers Bible*. New York: Wiley Publishing Inc. 1995. Print.

Chapter 8

1. Carter, James P. MD. *Racketeering In Medicine,* Virginia: Hampton Roads Publishing Company Inc., 1993. P. 40 Print.
2. " '20/20' Targets Chiropractic Pediatrics." (by the editorial staff). *Dynamic Chiropractic*. 25 Feb. 1994. Volume 12 Issue 5. Web. Accessed 2/2/2014. >http://www.dynamic chiropractic.com/mpacms/dc/article.php?id=41100<
3. Stephenson, Robert, DC, PHC. *The Chiropractic Textbook*. Vol. XII. Copyright 1927. Palmer School of Chiropractic.
4. Plank, Max. Lecture 'Das Wesen der Materie' [The Essential /Nature/Max-Character of Matter], Florence Italy (1944). Web Accessed 10/17/13. >http://todayinsci.com/P/Plank_Quotations.htm<
5. Glidden, Peter. *The MD Emperor Has No Clothes...Everybody Is sick And I Know Why*. United States: >www.drglidden.com.< No Publisher listed. P. 27 print.
6. American Medical Association Promoted Tobacco, Cigarettes in its Medical Journal. Smoking News Blog. April 20, 2011. Web. Accessed 12/18/2012. >http://www.smokersnews. net/american-medical-association-promoted-tobacco-cigarettes-<
7. Gardner, Martha N. PhD, Brandt, Allen M. PhD. *The Doctors' Choice Is America's Choice*. Am. Journal of Public Health. 2006 Febuary; 96(2): 222-232. Web. Accessed 1/14/14. >http:// www.ncbi.nlm.nih.gov/pmc/articles/PMC1470496/<
8. Report on Carcinogens, Twelfth Edition. National Institutes of Health (NEIHS). > http://ntp.neih.nih.gov/go/roc12<
9. "What's in a Cigarette?" American Lung Association. Web. Accessed 2/2/2015.

10. Hyman, Mark MD. *Ultrametabolism*. New York: Scribner, 2006. P. 24-25. Print.

Chapter 9

1. Senate Document #264. Better Health Thru Research. Web 26. Accessed 9/26/13. >http://betterhealththruresearch.com/document264htm.<
2. Concentrated Animal Feeding Operation: This is Animal Husbandry? >http://www3.factory-farming.com/CAFO.html<
3. Ponnampalam EN, Mann NJ, Sinclair AJ. "Effect of feeding systems on omega 3 fatty acids, conjugated linoleic acid and trans fatty acids in Australian beef cuts: potential impact on human health." *Asia Pacific Journal of Clinical Nutrition.* 2006;15(1):21-9. Pub Med. Department of Food Science, RMIT University, Melbourne, Victoria 3001, Austrailia.
4. Tsindos, Spero. "What drove us to drink 2 liters of water a day." *Austrailian and New Zealand Journal of Public Health.* 2012. Vol. 36 no.3 P.205-207.
5. Wallach, Joel, Ma Lan MD. *Immortality.* CA: Wellness Publications LLC, 2008. P. 2-4 Print.
6. Ibid. P. 84
7. 2010 Annual Report of the American Association of Poison Control Centers National Poison Data System (NPDS):28th Annual Report.
8. Mercola, Joe MD. "Over 60 Billion Doses a Year and Not ONE Death, but Still Not Safe? *Mercola.com*. Web. Accessed on 5/2/2012. >http://articles.mercola.com/sites/articles/archive/ 2012/04/23/defend-yo...<
9. Wallach, Joel, Ma Lan MD. *Rare Earths Forbidden Cures,* CA:Double Happiness Publishing Co., 1996. P. 167 Print.
10. Ibid. P. 25
11. Ibid. P. 251-263
12. Huff, Ethan A. "Organic Sulfur Study". Web. Accessed 5/5/2014. >http://cellular-oxygenation.com/Organic_Sulfur_Study.html.

13. Cancer, Sulfur, Garlic & Glutathione, Dr. Sircus. Web. Accessed on 11/23/2013. >http://drsircus.com/medicine/cancer/cancer-sulfur-garlic-glutathione<
14. Wallach, Joel, Ma Lan MD. *Rare Earths Forbidden Cures,* CA: Double Happiness Publishing Co. 1996. P. 19 Print.
15. Ibid. P. 53-58
16. Champagne, ET. "Low gastric hydrochloric acid secretion and mineral bioavailability." Pub Med. Adv Exp Med Biol., 1998;249:173-84. Web. Accessed on 11/27/2013. >http://www.ncbi.nlm.nih.org/pubmed/2543192<
17. Toscano, Amy. "Do Lentils Contain All Nine Essential Amino Acids?" Livestrong.com. Web. Accessed 1/27/2013. >http://www.livestrong.com/article/543944-do-lentils-contain-all-nine-essential-amino-acids/<
18. Ponnampalam EN, Mann NJ, Sinclair AJ. "Effect of feeding systems on omega-3 fatty acids, conjugated linoleic acid and trans fatty acids in Australian beef cuts: potential impact on human health." *Asia Pacific Journal of Clinical Nutrition.* 2006;15(1):21-9. Dept of food Science, RMIT University, Melbourne, Victoria 3001, Australia. PubMed.
19. Wallach, Joel. Ma Lan MD. *Rare Earths Forbidden Cures,* CA:Double Happiness Publishing Co., 1996. P. 379-382 Print.

Chapter 10
1. Wallach, Joel, Ma Lan MD. *Immortality.* CA: Wellness Publications LLC, 2008. Print.
2. Winter, Ruth MS. *A Consumers Dictionary of Food Additives.* New York: Three Rivers Press 1999. P. 358 Print.
3. Wallach, Joel ND. Ma Lan MD. *God Bless America.* CA: Wellness Publications L.L.C., 2013 Print. p.( ).

4. Sisson, Mark, *The Primal Blueprint*. California: Primal Nutrition Inc.2009. Print
5. Wikipedia, Negro Baseball League. Web, accessed on 6 Sept, 2013. >http://en.wikipedia.org/wiki/Negro_League_baseball<

Chapter 11

1. Locke, John. *How I Sold 1 Million e-Books in 5 Months*. Telemachus Press LLC, 2011.
2. Tolle, Eckhardt. *The Power of Now*. California: New World Library, 2004. Print.
3. Dyer, Wayne. *Your Erroneous Zones*. New York: Quill, 2001. Print. Originally published by Harper Collins in 1991.
4. Chopra, Depak MD. *What Are You Hungry For*. New York: Harmony Books, 2013. P.12. Print
5. Hyman, Mark MD. *Ultrametabolism*. New York: Scribner, 2006. P. 15-16 Print.
6. Cloud, Henry, John Townsend. *Boundaries*. USA: Yates and Yates, 1992. Print.
7. Sharma, Robin. *Who Will Cry When You Die*. California: Hay House, 2002. Print. Originally published by Harper Collins 1999.
8. Sharma, Robin. *The Monk Who Sold His Ferrari*. San Fransisco: Harper Collins, 1997. Print.
9. Dyer, Wayne. *Getting in The Gap*. California: Hay House, 2003. Print
10. Truman, Carol. *Feelings Buried Alive Never Die*. Utah: Olympus Distributing, 2003. Print.
11. Dyer, Wayne. *There's A Spiritual Solution To Every Problem*. New York: Quill, 2003. Print.
12. Young, Robert O. *The pH Miracle*. New York: Wellness Central (Hachette Book Group), 2010.
13. Ibid. P. 22-24

14. Ibid. P. 29-49
15. Free Radicals. Wikipedia. Web. Accessed 1/15/14. >http://en.wikipedia.org/wiki/Radical_(chemistry)<
16. Wallach, Joel, Ma Lan MD. *Immortality.* CA: Wellness Publications LLC, 2008. P. 31 Print.
17. Morgan, Graeme, Robyn Ward, Michael Barton. "The Contribution of Cytotoxic Chemotherapy to 5-Year Survival in Adult Malignancies." *Clinical Oncology* (2004) 16:549-560.
18. The Raw Milk Movement: Healthy of Hazardous? A Campaign for Real Milk. Web. Accessed 6/30/2014. >http://www.realmilk.com/safety/raw-milk-movement-healthy-or-hazardous/<
19. Ibid.
20. Ibid.
21. Ibid.
22. Fallon, Sally. *Nourishing Traditions.* Washington DC: New Trends Publishing Inc., 2005. P.33-34. Print.

Index

A
Aborigines, 166
Abraham Flexner, 12
acesulfame-K, 118, 205
acid reflux, 35, 47
acidic, 185
acidosis, 185
acne, 47,
acrylamide, 120
ADD, 68
adderall, 68
ADHD, 56, 68, 123
adrenal exhaustion, 145
aflatoxins, 107
agave, 80, 117
Agent Orange, 125
agrichemicals, 39
air fresheners, 128
Albert Einstein, 15
ALCAT test, 52, 55

alcohol, 65, 189
alkaline, 39
alkalinity, 186
allergies, 53, 57, 146, 158, 187
allopathy, 10
almonds, 107
ALS, (see Lou Gehrig's disease)
Alzheimer's disease, 2, 5, 14, 83, 102, 109, 115, 152
amino acids, 51, 78, 156, 160, 170
Amino-Sweet, 64
anaphylaxis, 55
Ancel Keys, 91
Andrew Still DO., 13
anemia (iron deviciency), 155
    pernicious, 155
anthocyanins, 77
anti-inflammatory drugs, 52
anti-nutrients, 63

• 257

antioxidants, 77, 79, 101, 189
anxiety, 55, 56, 115, 123
aortic aneurysm, 15,
apricot seeds (laetrile), 107
arrythmias, 115
arthritis, 15, 30, 31, 47, 53, 70, 86, 158
aspartame, 36, 114, 115, 205
aspartic acid, 114
asthma, 30, 47, 53, 55, 130, 158
attitude, 178
autism, 56
autolyzed yeast, 109

B
B-17 (laetrile), 107
Back pain, 139, 142
bad breath, 70
balance, 199
barley, 57
barley malt syrup, 80
Barry Sears, 23
beans, 212
bee pollen, 68
beef tallow, 88
benzine, 118
benzidine, 122
beriberi, 155
berries, 204
Berkey filters, 38
biochemical individuality, 4, 20

bi-polar disorder, 56
birth defects, 23
bison meat, 104, 161
Bisphenol-A (BPA), 111, 132, 201, 207
bleaching, 87
blindness, 115
bloating, 55
blood, 28
bloody stool, 55
blue # 2,
blurred vision, 115, 123
body care products, 27, 135
bone loss, 35
bottled water, 40
boullion, 109, 206
Bovine Growth Hormone (rBGH), 192
bowel function, 51
brain fog, 145
breast milk, 191
Brominated Vegetable Oil, (BVO), 112
    cash register reciepts, 111
bromine, 112
brown rice syrup, 80
Bt-toxin, 56
butter, 101, 192, 208
bypass surgery, 92, 155

C

caffeine, 1, 154, 160
calcium, 35, 144, 155, 156, 193
calcium caseinate, 109
calorie restricted diets, 166
cancer, 14, 41, 53, 71, 86, 95, 99, 123, 128, 136, 147, 152, 158, 187, 200
    DNA coding and cancer, 187
    Malignant cancer treatment, 190
    Ovarian cancer and talcum powder, 134
Canadian Football League, 175
Canderel, 114
candidiasis, 53
canola oil, 87
carbohydrate, 62
carcinogens, 108, 118, 121, 127, 131, 122
cardiomyopathy, 168
cardiovascular disease, 14,
Celiac disease, 46, 47, 53, 54, 56, 58
cereals, 43, 48
chemicals,
chemotherapy, 128, 155, 190
Chinese restaurant syndrome, 109
chiropractic, 27, 137, 143
chlorine, 38
chocolate (dark), 206
cholesterol, 82, 89, 91, 92, 101, 102, 163, 204
    low cholesterol, 95
chromium, 34, 36, 163
chronic fatigue syndrome, 53, 115
chronic obstructive pulmonary disease (COPD), 152
cigarettes, 73, 146,
    chemicals in, 147
cinnamon, 163
citrus red # 2, 123
cleaning supplies, 129, 130
coconut oil, 88, 102
Co-enzyme Q-10, 162
co-factors, 36
coffee, 33, 37, 121, 205
coffee creamers, 100
connective tissue disorders. 158
complex sugars (carbohydrates), 74, 77
concentrated animal feeding operations, (CAFO), 152
constipation, 30, 33, 53, 70
contact dermatitis, 131
copper, 15
corn, 90
corn oil, 83, 87
coronary heart disease, 77
cosmetics, 27,
cotton seed oils, 87, 88

C-reactive protein, 106
cribbing, 159
Crisco, 83
Crohn's disease, 46, 53, 58
cruciferous vegetables, 78
curry, 190
cystoic acid, 110

D
D. D. Palmer, 137
DNA coding (cancer), 187
date sugars, 80
death certificates, 94
deer meat (venison), 161
degenerative joint disease, 31
dehydration, 33, 63, 142, 146
dental cavities, 84
deodorization, 87
depression, 24, 53, 95, 115, 123
desmosomes, 51
diabetes, 1, 2, 14, 47, 53, 55, 86, 96, 152, 187
    Type 3 diabetes, 102
diaper rash, 55
diarrhea, 53, 55, 70, 123
diet, 23
diet drinks, 100,
diet- heart hypothesis, 98
dioxane (1-4), 131
disaccharides, 62
disc herniations, 147
dizziness, 130
donuts, 48, 49
dry mouth, 30
dysbiosis, 53

E
early puberty, 111
eclectic medicine, 10, 11
eczema, 47, 54
egg substitutes, 195
eggs, 101, 158, 203
Einkorn wheat, 57
electrolytes, 42
Emmer wheat, 57
emotional eating, 179
emotional stress, 180
endocrine disruption, 41, 127
endometriosis, 89
energy drinks, 33
enlarged prostate, 111
enriched breads, 45, 195
environmental chemicals, 185
enzymes, 78, 139
EPA/DHA, 106, 107, 161
epilepsy, 115
Epstein-Barr, 115
Equal, 114
erectile dysfunction (ED), 89, 102
erythritol, 117
essential fatty acids, 156, 201
esterified rosin, 112

excitotoxin, 109
excretion, 30
exercise, 164, 167, 172, 174
extrusion, 58

F
fats, 82
fatty acids, 101, 106, 170 (see Omega 3, 6, 9 oils)
fatigue, 30, 47, 115, 145, 187
fiber, 78
fibromyalgia, 15, 30, 47, 53, 70, 86,
fight or flight, 31, 167, 180
fingernail polish, 126
flax seed oil, 89
Flexner Report, 11
fluoride, 38
folic acid, 190
food additives, 105, 185
food allergies, 46, 52, 68, 69, 146, 187
food colorings, 68, 121- 123, 160
food cravings, 53
food labels, 193
food sensitivities, 69
forgiveness, 184
formaldehyde, 114, 130
formic acid, 114
free glutamic acid, 108, 109, 110
free radicals, 189

free range eggs, 64, 97, 164, 203, 204
free range meats, 161
French fries, 121
fructose, 67
fungicides, 44, 58

G
GALT, 51
GAPS diet, 68
garlic, 158
gas, 55
Gatorade, 112, 169
genetics, 20, 23, 148
genetic modification, 79 , 87, 201
George Washington, 11
glacier runoff, 166
gliadin, 44
glucose, 67
glutamic acid, 109
gluten, 56, 57
GMO corn, 56
goals, 176
good bacteria (gut), 50
gout, 70
grass fed beef, 103
gray hair,
gut flora,

H
hair dyes, 126

hair-spray, 135
Harvard Food Plate, 55
headaches, 30, 55, 115, 123, 130
health care, 25
Health Pyramid, 22
hearing loss, 115
heart attacks, 83, 147, 168
heart disease, 5, 86, 92, 99, 105, 111, 152
    heart disease costs, 97
heart palpitations, 123
heavy metals, 38, 39
hemorrhoids, 15
hemp oil, 89, 106
herbicides, 39, 88
heterocyclic amines, 200
Hering's Law of Cure, 141
high fructose corn syrup, 35, 62, 67, 71, 78
hip replacements, 147
Hippocrates, 137
hives, 54, 123
homeopathy, 10
homeostasis, 28
homocysteine, 106
honey, 67, 204
hormone disrupters, 108
hospitals, 12, 15, 64, 100, 116
hot dogs, 111
Huntington's disease, 109
Hunza's, 165

hybridization, 43, 58, 87, 196
hydration, 29, 42
hydrogen potential, 185
hydrogenated fats, 46, 83, 86, 87, 101, 192
hydrogenated spreads, 87, 100
hydrolyzed protein, 109, 110, 206, 209
hyperactivity, 115
hypercholesterolemia, 106
hypertension, 5, 30, 53, 70, 140
hypothyroidism, 115

I

IgG-4, 52
immunity, 51, 53
infections, 7, 50, 51, 109, 132
inflammation, 31, 47, 48, 67, 77, 92, 97, 105, 160
innate intelligence, 138, 139, 142
insecticides, 44
insomnia, 30, 47, 53, 115
insulin, 47, 67, 80, 104, 139
intestinal flora, 51
intestinal permeability, 57
irregular menstrual cycles, 89
irritability, 55
irritable bowel syndrome (IBS), 47, 53, 70
isomalt, 117
itching, 123

J
joint pain, 115
junk foods, 3, 24, 71, 86, 91, 92, 106, 120, 162

K
Kangen water, 39
ketosis, 186
ketogenic diet, 186, 189
kidney problems, 187
knee replacements, 155
krill, 107

L
lacitol, 117
lard, 88, 103
LDL cholesterol, 104, 105
leaky gut syndrome, 50
learning disabilities, 68, 111
leavening agents, 46
lemons, 37
lifestyle, 24
limes, 37
lipid-hypothesis, 91
lipstick, 135
lipoprotein-a, 106
liver problems, 41, 111
longevity, 14
Lou Gehrig's disease (ALS), 109, 115
love, 184
low-"T", 102
lupus, 15, 53
lye, 130
Lyme's Disease, 115
lymphoma, 55

M
Macadamia nuts, 161
make-up, 135
malabsorption, 46, 54, 160, 167
maltitol, 117
mannitol, 117
maple syrup, 67, 69, 204
margarine, 151, 192
mascara, 135
massage therapy, 144
mayonnaise, 210
Max Plank, 138, 139
Mazola, 83
meditation, 144
Mediterranean diet, 100, 213
memory Loss, 115
Menieres' Disease, 115
methanol, 114, 118
microfold cells, 51
migraine headaches, 89, 117
milk, 191,
minerals, 78, 79, 101, 152, 155, 156, 163, 170
mitochondrial disease, 181

mitochondrial function, 181
molds, 107
monoliasis, 53
monosaccharides, 62
monosodium glutamate (MSG), 64, 109, 192, 207, 208
mood disorders, 115, 187
motivation, 16,
multiple sclerosis (MS), 14, 53, 115, 136
MSM (sulfur), 159
multiple myeloma, 116
muscle cramps, 115
muscle weakness, 143 m
mustard, 210

N
nail polish, 135
natural flavor, 109, 110, 208
naturopathy, 10,
nausea, 115
neruotoxin, 127
neurological disease, 47, 53, 86, 114
NFL, (Pro football), 14
Nicoyan's, 165
nitrates, 111
nitrites, 111
nitrogen, 44
nitrosamines, 200
non-Hodgkin's lymphoma, 54, 126

numbness, 115
Nutra-Sweet, 36
nutritionists, 47, 48, 53, 65, 70, 76, 103, 156
nuts, 107, 158, 208
nut butters, 107
Nystatin, 53

O
oats, 59
obesity, 47, 53, 55, 86, 111, 140, 147, 149
oils, 82
Olestra, 65
oligosaccharides, 62
olive oil, 88, 102, 161
omega 3 fats, 161
omega 6 fats, 161
omega 9 fats, 161
oncologists, 188
onions, 158
ORAC points, 189
organ dysfunction, 143
osteoarthritis, 33,
osteopaths, 13
osteopathy, 10,
osteoporosis, 35, 54, 187
ovarian cancer, 134
ovarian dysfunction, 111
oven cleaners, 130

P

pain, 139, 143
    chronic, 140
pancreatic cancer, 55
parabens, 1332
Parkinson's disease, 14, 109, 136
pasta, 36, 43, 46, 48, 188, 202
peanuts, 208
pecans, 107, 208
peripheral neuropathies, 5, 55
persistent organic pollutants (POP's), 125
pesticides, 39, 58, 88
Peyer's patches, 51
pH, 38,
phenylalanine, 114
phenylketonuria, 114
phosphates, 129, 130
phosphorous, 35
phytates, 57, 107, 160, 167
phytic acid, 57, 107
phytonutrients, 77
pica, 159
pistachios, 107
plantar fasciitis, 173
plastic ID codes,
plasticization of fats, 87
plastics, 40
PMS, 89, 115
poached eggs, 101
poison, 114, 129
polycystic ovarian syndrome, 189
polyethelene terephthalate (PETE), 40
polypropylene (PP), 41
polyunsaturated fatty acid, (PUFA's), 59, 98, 102
popcorn, 121
Positron Emission Tomography (PET), 71
post-polio syndrome, 115
potassium, 44, 112, 156
Powerade, 113, 169
prayer, 9, 184
preservatives, 2, 15, 24, 64, 86, 111, 126, 132, 196, 215
processed foods, 97
processed wheat, 97
prostate cancer, 111
protein, 101
prudent diet, 18, 55, 59, 79, 97, 98, 152
psoriasis, 47

Q

quercetin, 190

R

rancid fat, 86, 97, 189
rashes, 130
raw milk, 88, 192

recumbinant Bovine Growth Hormone (rBGH), 192
red # 40,
refined carbohydrates, 71, 78
refined flour, 45, 91
refined oils, 87
refined sugar, 91
resin ID codes , 40, 41
respiration, 71
resveratrol, 190
reverse osmosis, 40
rheumatoid arthritis, 55
rice, 90
rickets, 155
Ritalin, 68
road rage, 24
Robert Stephenson DC., 138
Round Up, 87
rye, 57, 202

S
salmon, 107, 161
sardines, 107
saturated fat, 78, 98, 102, 105
schizophrenia, 56, 112
scoliosis, 32
Scott v. FDA, 119, 122
scurvy, 155
sea salt, 210, 211
secretory IgA, 50
seizures, 117, 189
selenium, 162, 168, 189
serotonin, 56
sex hormones, 101
simple sugar, 62
skin lesions, 115
skin problems, 30, 47, 52, 53, 70, 117, 158
sleep disturbance, 123
slurred speech, 115
small intestine, 50, 51, 52, 185
smoking, 24, 57, 74, 91, 97, 105, 146, 189
sodium lauryl sulfate, 131
soft drinks, 2, 20, 42, 29, 32-35, 61, 63, 65, 100, 106, 112, 120, 160
sorbitol, 117
soy milk, 209
soy oil, 87
spinal adjustments, 139
spinal cord, 143
Splenda, (see sucralose)
sports drinks, 33
SSRI's (serotonin re-uptake inhibitors), 56
Standard American Diet (SAD), 7, 65, 106, 155, 168, 185
statin drugs, 95, 96, 102
stevia, 37, 42, 80, 120, 204
stress, 24, 97 , 106, 180, 189
stiffness, 140

stints, 92
stroke, 91, 147, 152
sucralose, 116, 205
sugar, 3, 61, 105, 204
sugar alcohols, 117
suicide, 95
sulfur, 158, 159, 163, 203
surfactants, 129

T
Tai Chi, 172, 175
talcum powder, 128
tantrums, 55
tea, 33, 37
temperature, 144
textured protein, 109
The Delaney Clause, 118, 119, 122
The Flexner report, 10, 11
The Framingham study, 93
The French Paradox, 101
The glycemic index, 45, 75
thyroid function, 146
tinnitus, 70, 115
topsoil, 90
Tourette's syndrome, 56
toxins, 25, 108
toxic burden, 27
trauma, 25
triglycerides, 67, 97, 104
triticum aestivum (wheat), 43, 47

turbinado sugar, 80
turmeric, 190
tuna, 161
TV dinners, 73, 109, 110, 196, 206

U
ulcerative colitis, 46, 53
ulcers, 77
USDA food pyramid, 18, 55, 102

V
vanadium, 34, 36, 163
varicose veins, 15,
vegetables (non starchy), 74, 77, 78, 80, 97, 103, 164, 186, 190, 200, 216
venison, 102, 104, 161
vertigo, 115
veterinarians, 15, 93
Viet-Nam, 13, 125
Vilacabamban's, 165
villi, 50
Vioxx, 44
vitalism, 138
vital nerve energy, 143
vitamins, 51, 78, 101, 155, 156, 160, 170
vitamin A, 189
vitamin deficiency, 146
vitamin C, 155, 163, 189, 190

vitamin E, 168, 189
volatile organic compounds
  (VOC's), 130
vomiting, 123

W
walnuts, 107
water, 29 , 153 , 154
WD 40, 136
weight gain, 117, 187
Weston A. Price Foundation, 84
White, Paul Ducley, MD., 83
wheat, 31, 43, 90, 104
wheat allergy, 46
wheat sensitivities, 46
wheezing, 55
wood ashes, 157
wrinkles, 15,

X
xenoestrogens, 41
xylitol, 117

Y
yeast, 50
yeast infections, 52
yeast overgrowth, 53
yeast problems, 52, 53
yellow # 5 (Tartraine), 121, 122
yellow # 6 (Sunset Yellow), 121, 122
yoga, 144, 175

Z
zinc, 163

CPSIA information can be obtained
at www.ICGtesting.com
Printed in the USA
FSHW021327311020
75343FS